VOICE CARE

IN THE
MEDICAL SETTING

The completion of this book was a labor of love and loneliness. To say we lost one of the world's best clinicians on November 17th, 1994, would be to greatly understate Danna's remarkable legacy. The sensitivity, dedication, and thoroughness with which she undertook every personal, clinical, and academic task was extraordinary. Her infallible sense of principle guided her at every moment and inspired her patients, colleagues, students, and friends. Her genuine concern for others earned the trust and respect of all those who had the pleasure of interacting with her. Danna's optimistic outlook, her vibrant love of life, and her beautiful smile brought sunshine to our lives on the cloudiest days. She leaves behind many forlorn friends, family members, colleagues, and patients. Fortunately, she also leaves the legacy of her wisdom, experience, and clinical talents between the covers of this book. We thank you Danna.

VOICE CARE
IN THE
MEDICAL SETTING

Danna Loeh Koschkee, M.A.
Department of Surgery
University of Wisconsin Hospital and Clinics
Madison, Wisconsin

with

Linda Rammage, Ph.D.
Department of Surgery
The University of British Columbia
Vancouver, Canada

To Del:

Thanks for your support and friendship

Linda

SINGULAR PUBLISHING GROUP, INC.
SAN DIEGO · LONDON

Singular Publishing Group, Inc.
401 West "A" Street, Suite 325
San Diego, California 92101-7904

Singular Publishing Group, Ltd.
19 Compton Terrace
London, N1 2UN, UK

e-mail: singpub@mail.cerfnet.com
Website: http://www.singpub.com

Typeset in 10/12 Palatino by So Cal Graphics
Printed in the United States of America by McNaughton and Gunn

Library of Congress Cataloging-in-Publication Data

Koschkee, Danna Loeh.
  Voice care in the medical setting / by Danna Loeh Koschkee ; with
Linda Rammage.
      p.   cm.
  Includes bibliographical references and index.
  ISBN 1–56593–111–4
  1. Voice disorders.   I. Rammage, Linda.   II. Title.
  [DNLM: 1. Voice Disorders—diagnosis.   2. Voice Disorders—
therapy.   WV 500 K86v 1997]
  RF510.K67   1997
  616.85'5—dc21
  DNLM/DLC`
  for Library of Congress   97–11209
                                                                     CIP

CONTENTS

FOREWORD

"Challenging" accurately describes the problem facing vocologists attempting to assess and treat persons with voice disorders. Vocologists' present-day accomplishments in caring for patients with voice deficits have been ably assisted by parallel developments in several medically related fields, the performing arts, and technology. In the following text, Danna Koschkee, along with Linda Rammage, share their collective experiences obtained in clinical care at both the University of Wisconsin and Vancouver Hospital. The book will serve as the reference standard for years to come, as it easily accomplishes its main goal—to aid clinicians in their interdisciplinary efforts to understand the problems faced and the solutions proposed in voice care in the medical setting.

Koschkee's main theme, simply stated, is that diagnosis and treatment of voice disorders must be studied as an aggregate—a collective and integrative unity of fields such as otolaryngology, psychology, and speech pathology, of science and art, and of individual occupational, emotional, and social needs. Reiterated throughout the text is the author's commitment to the notion that voice care requires a wedding of medical terminology with clinical practice, that voice care should be carried out by knowledgeable clinicians working in an interdisciplinary environment, and further that clinicians must apply in an artful manner scientific principles to the care of individuals with voice disorders. The merging of art and science and the blurring between the lines traditionally thought to separate the two appear to serve as the underlying philosophy of voice care in the medical setting. The author consistently draws examples from everyday practices in hospital settings to underscore this philosophy and clarify her points of emphasis. From developing a laboratory to taking a case history to planning and monitoring treatment, she demonstrates how scientific principles of hypothesis development and the art of careful scientific observation can be applied to better serve the voice disordered patient. Here, Danna's and Linda's rich background as voice clinicians permits them to link current theories of practice with the demanding problems faced daily by clinicians working in the clinical trenches. The book deals not only with tough clinical issues but also with problems associated with developing and maintaining a program in a time of ever diminishing resources and increasing workloads.

As a fellow voice clinician, I have shared Danna Koschkee's and Linda Rammage's beliefs that integration of information from a good case history and interpretation of instrumental measures obtained during vocal gymnastics hold promise for unraveling some of the mysteries of voice disorders that have continued to escape our understanding. As a professional peer, I too have observed that the sum of the interdisciplinary parts offered by speech pathologists, otolaryngologists, psychiatrists, neurologists, endocrinologists, pulmonologists, singing teachers, and vocal coaches is much greater than the individual parts. As a vocal educator, I have been most sympathetic with their desire to incorporate the knowledge derived from these observations into the mainstream of thought of vocology. Consequently, I view it as a privilege to write this brief foreword to *Voice Care in the Medical Setting*. I mark the occasion as one in which a long-needed and timely publication takes its place in the literature on training of vocologists and care of individuals with voice disorders in a medical setting.

My only regret in writing this foreword is that Danna Koschkee did not live to see the book in print. She would be proud of the finished product brought to fruition by her close friend and colleague. Danna's creative mind, enthusiasm, and work in the interest of persons with voice disorders served as an inspiration to those who knew her. Now others can also share in this rich legacy by reading her book, written with Linda Rammage, on *Voice Care in the Medical Setting*, and putting the knowledge into practice.

Diane M. Bless, Ph.D.
Madison, Wisconsin

PREFACE

Voice care in the medical setting is a multidisciplinary endeavor that has evolved over the past two decades into a specialty practice: a specialty practice that is defined by our current understanding of vocal anatomy and physiology, state-of-the-art technology, and refined medical-surgical and therapeutic techniques.

Recent major advancements in science and technology impacting on medical practices have necessitated that a more sophisticated level of training and skills be acquired by those involved in management of persons with voice disorders. The wide variety of etiological bases for voice disorders dictates the need for multidisciplinary collaboration among medical practitioners from a variety of specialty disciplines. As we advance into the 21st century, the voice care team needs to acknowledge and take advantage of technologies that facilitate the most effective and accurate medical management, while simultaneously nurturing the "human" role, by developing those clinical skills that only perceptive, knowledgeable, sensitive and well-trained clinicians can offer. All of these requirements must be met for optimal practice of voice care, with the added challenge of a political and economic climate that dictates restraint at both corporate and individual practitioner levels. Modern voice clinicians need to be as-

tute clinic managers, to advocate for the best standards of care on behalf of the population they serve and to ensure the clinical voice program functions effectively within administrative and budgetary guidelines.

Voice Care in the Medical Setting was prepared for clinicians from a variety of disciplines who work together to provide assessment, diagnostic, and treatment services for individuals with voice disorders. Both the scientific-technological issues impacting on modern clinical voice laboratories and key aspects of multidisciplinary clinical management are addressed in detail. For the newly formed voice care team, the text provides comprehensive information regarding history-taking, formal and informal observational assessment methods, instrumental voice evaluation, interdisciplinary referral, current trends in treatment, and program planning and expansion. For the student-clinician or new clinician entering the specialty arena, procedural guidelines for assessment, diagnosis, treatment, and treatment efficacy evaluation are provided, generously complemented with procedural flow-charts, clinical forms and protocols, and descriptive tables. For clinical administrators planning an interdisciplinary voice clinic, the book is a resource for defining the current status of voice care technology and care and program-planning details such as space requirements, staffing requirements, professional roles and relationships, and reporting and billing procedures.

The management techniques described in this text reflect an international perspective. References and clinical protocols are represented that were developed in many different centers of excellence around the world. The contemporary clinician needs access to a pool of international resources in such a rapidly growing medical specialty field as voice care. We hope clinicians and their patients can benefit from this global knowledge base as we strive to offer the best voice care possible in centers around the world.

ACKNOWLEDGMENTS

To our families, friends, colleagues, and employers who supported the completion of this book: please accept our deepest thanks. Special thanks to our mentor, Diane Bless, for her constant moral and academic support. We are grateful to Celeste Kirk and Dr. Mark Leddy for their invaluable editorial efforts and suggestions. Thanks also to Dr. Murray Morrison, Dr. Christy Ludlow, Dr. Douglas Graeb, Dr. Charles Ford, and Dr. James Brandenburg for their helpful contributions.

So many people: colleagues, teachers, parents, clients, and friends have inspired and influenced the philosophies and knowledge base that are reflected in these chapters, that it is difficult to provide a suitably comprehensive acknowledgment. Let us conclude by thanking the many health care pioneers of yesterday, today, and tomorrow, who, with courage and dedication, have continued to explore and define better ways to provide effective health care to our fellow humans.

On Danna's behalf, I dedicate this work to her family: Jim, Jeffrey, Corinne, Sandy, Betty, Rodney, Jack, Bill, the nieces and nephews she adored, and the memory of Rick. You know how much Danna loved you.

Linda

CHAPTER

1

VOICE CARE

Wedding Medical Technology with Clinical Practice

Voice care in the medical setting today is a wedding of medical technology and clinical practice. It is necessarily a marriage of science and art, instrument and heart. The skills and talents involved in delivering voice care—detecting the presence of laryngeal anomalies, applying objective diagnostic tests, assessing subjective manifestations of voice production, synthesizing test results, and designing voice treatment protocols—embrace all the knowledge and experience health care professionals can offer. These skills and abilities are now being revolutionized by remarkable changes in technology.

For speech pathologists, changes in technology have dramatically altered their roles in delivering voice care. They now have access to powerful equipment and instrumentation that contribute enormously to the diagnosis and treatment of vocal pathologies. Because of their clinical expertise in using these diagnostic and assessment tools, and their comprehensive understanding of nor-

mal and abnormal phonatory physiology, speech pathologists have become integral members of medical teams.

For laryngologists, technological advancements in voice assessment and surgical techniques have enhanced the evaluation process and changed the goals of surgery (Ford & Bless, 1991). As stronger relationships with other voice specialists develop and phonosurgery comes of age, new opportunities for maximizing patient care are emerging.

Now more than ever, voice care professionals—speech pathologists, laryngologists, singing and drama coaches, psychiatrists, psychologists, allergists, pulmonologists, endocrinologists, and neurologists—are coming together, in research, in clinics, in surgery, and in therapy, employing the new technologies to provide interdisciplinary care to patients with the full array of laryngeal disorders. This union has opened new vistas for diagnosing and treating conditions related to head and neck tumors, vocal abuse and misuse, metabolic laryngeal dysfunctions, granulomatous laryngeal disease, rheumatologic voice disorders, reflux laryngitis, vocal fold paralysis, psychogenic voice disorders, inflammatory laryngeal diseases, congenital abnormalities of the larynx, neurologic voice disorders, voice problems related to gender dysphoria, toxicogenic dysphonias, and changes in the larynx due to the aging process.

Tremendous benefits have been afforded to patients as a result of this interdisciplinary approach to voice care. A higher standard of practice is now possible because professionals are collaborating in the assessment of the incoming patient, coordinating their diagnostic and treatment efforts, committing themselves as members of a voice care team, and sharing the responsibility for establishing a proper, well-monitored therapy program.

With these advances in mind, the elements that comprise a comprehensive, sensitive, technologically sound voice care program are presented in this book. Technology has created this new view of voice care in a new age, but goals related to patients' well-being remain the focus of every effort.

TECHNOLOGY AS AN AGENT OF CHANGE

The impact of the wedding between medical technology and clinical practice has changed five major aspects of voice care:

▶ Diagnostic techniques,
▶ Assessment methodologies,
▶ Treatment approaches and procedures,
▶ Professional roles and relationships, and
▶ Cost of services.

The first four of these changes have, in turn, engendered new benefits for patients and their families.

Advances in Diagnostic Techniques

Advances in the diagnosis of voice disorders have progressed rapidly since 1970. An era distinguished by "high-technology" breakthroughs, innovative research, and interdisciplinary collaboration originated in the 1970s and gained momentum during the following two decades. Newer technologies in the subspecialties of *diagnostic imaging* and *clinical examinations of voice* have revolutionized voice diagnostic programs, enabling practitioners to become more accountable and improving their ability to relate structure and function to the sound of the voice.

Diagnostic Imaging

In the 1970s and 1980s, five major diagnostic imaging procedures were introduced to voice care professionals: magnetic resonance imaging, computed tomography, ultrasonography, videofluoroscopy, and videostroboscopy. These imaging advances are discussed in detail in Chapter 4, but are briefly introduced in this chapter to set the stage for discussing the impact of technology on medical voice care.

Magnetic Resonance Imaging: Considered by many to be the most important medical imaging advance of the century, magnetic resonance imaging (MRI) has proven to be an invaluable diagnostic tool in the assessment of head and neck lesions. Since its inception over 20 years ago, MRI has evolved to become the imaging modality of choice in the evaluation of most central nervous system and spinal disorders (Mafee, Langer, Valvassori, Soboroff, & Friedman, 1986). Through MR scanning, it has become possible to visualize the soft tissue structures of the head and neck in exquisite detail. Two- and three-dimensional images of the head and neck regions are used to detect and diagnose a variety of abnormalities including central nervous system disorders (e.g., Parkinson's disease), neuromuscular diseases (e.g., myasthenia gravis), and head or neck tumors (e.g., laryngeal cancer).

Computed Tomography: Despite the advantages of MRI as a neurophysiological diagnostic aid, conventional imaging (plain films) and computed tomography (CT) continue to be the foundation of otolaryngologic imaging (Unger, 1987). Whereas plain films image only hard tissues and MRI images only soft tissues, CT offers visualization of both soft and hard tissues. Consequently, the CT scan can provide incomparable diagnostic information to the laryngologist during preoperative assessments of patients with head and neck tumors (Kuhns, Thornburg, & Fryback, 1989) and of individuals with acute laryngeal trauma (Schaeffer, 1991).

Ultrasonography: Although ultrasound has been used most commonly for assessing pathologic conditions involving organs such as the thyroid, heart, and bladder, and in demonstrating fetal movements, this technology can also offer valuable diagnostic information about the larynx and phonatory function (Bohme, 1989). When used to assess the larynx, the high-frequency sound waves yield images of the position, form, and function of laryngeal structures at the infraglottic, glottic, and supraglottic levels. Ultrasonography is used primarily in assessing the larynges of infants and children, since the higher density and thickness of an adult's thyroid lamina can potentially prevent effective visualization. Because of its noninvasiveness, its application to the pediatric population, and its ability to image infraglottal structures, this technology provides unique diagnostic information.

Videofluoroscopy: Recently, videofluoroscopy has found wide application in the assessment of swallowing and voice disorders. Swallowing studies (modified barium swallow or modified barium swallow plus esophagram) are used routinely to identify structural, physiological, and behavioral problems associated with swallowing (Edberg, 1992). In addition, videofluoroscopic testing can aid in assessing velopharyngeal dysfunction (McWilliams, Morris, & Shelton, 1990), glottic incompetence (Colton & Casper, 1990), and alaryngeal voice problems such as hyperconstriction of the upper esophageal segment or improper placement of a tracheo-esophageal prosthesis (Sloane, Griffin, & O'Dwyer, 1991). The clinical usefulness of videofluoroscopy, particularly in the assessment of swallowing

disorders, is reflected in the high accessibility of this diagnostic tool, available in most hospitals today.

Videostroboscopy: Although stroboscopy was first used in 1878, clinical application to laryngeal imaging did not develop until a century later. Since the 1970s, videostroboscopy has become an established diagnostic procedure for assessing the entire spectrum of laryngeal pathologies (Hirano & Bless, 1993).

Classical endoscopy (visual inspection of the larynx using an endoscope and constant light source) allows practitioners to examine the vocal folds and related structures. Videostroboscopy (stroboscopic light source and video recording equipment coupled with the endoscope) provides additional, critical information about vocal fold vibration. Consequently, the technique of videostroboscopy combines a thorough examination of the laryngeal structures, and vibratory patterns exhibited during phonation.

The diagnostic value of stroboscopy has been well documented (Woo, Colton, Casper, & Brewer, 1991; Bless, Hirano, & Feder, 1987, and others). In their study of patients with hoarse voices, Woo et al. (1991) found that videostroboscopic examinations contributed significant diagnostic information more than 25% of the time; following videostroboscopic testing, diagnoses were changed in 15 patients: for 6, surgery was avoided; for 9, surgery was indicated in lieu of voice and/or medical therapy.

Clinical Examinations of Voice

Other types of clinical examinations of voice—critical elements of the assessment process—have also been altered by technological developments. These tests include assessments of phonatory ability and laryngeal movement, observational-perceptual, aerodynamic, and acoustic evaluations (vocal function analysis), and electromyography (electrophysiological analysis). These assessment protocols, discussed further in Chapters 3 and 4, represent the classical modes of voice pathology diagnosis.

Analysis of Vocal Function: During vocal function testing, the speech pathologist administers a comprehensive battery of tests designed to evaluate respiratory, phonatory, and resonatory function. This diagnostic battery includes both instrumental and noninstrumental examinations of voice. Objective, instrumental measures (e.g., fundamental frequency, frequency range, intensity, intensity range, airflow rate, glottal resistance, vital capacity, nasalance) are obtained using sophisticated, biomedical laboratory equipment. The Nagashima Phonatory Function Analyzer (Kelleher Medical, Inc., Richmond, VA); C-Speech Software (Milenkovic, Madison, WI); the Nasometer (Kay Elemetrics Corp, Pine Brook, NJ); IBM Personal System/2 Speechviewer (IBM National Support Center for Persons with Disabilities, Atlanta, GA); the Laryngograph (Kay Elemetrics Corp., Pine Brook, NJ); and Respitrace (Ambulatory Monitoring, Inc., Ardsley, NY) are among the dedicated physiological data acquisition and analysis systems that can generate objective vocal function data.

The observational-perceptual assessment encompasses a wide range of formal and informal clinical activities leading to judgments of the nature and degree of observable features associated with a voice disorder. This assessment is conducted via visual, auditory, or tactile-kinesthetic perceptions. Auditory-perceptual rating scales are used to describe and quantify the perceptual characteristics of voice, although most assess only cursory features of phonation (e.g., pitch, loudness, and quality). Other scales, such as the Vocal Profile Analysis system (Laver & MacKenzie-Beck, 1991) delve comprehensively into the intricacies of voice production as they relate to the entire vocal tract, including the supraglottic resonators (e.g., lip, tongue, jaw, and velopharyngeal positioning). Used together, these two types of instrumental and scaling techniques for auditory-perceptual analysis allow clinicians to separate respiratory from resonatory and laryngeal function, to profile patients' unique phonatory patterns, and to assist in determining the pathogenesis of dysphonias. Furthermore, these techniques provide objective documentation supporting the efficacy of surgical, medical, and behavioral treatments.

Visual-perceptual and tactile-perceptual observation of general and speech-related postures are used to specify areas and degrees of muscle use and misuse associated with speech and vocalizing in individuals with voice disorders. Although most clinicians use subjective nonstandardized judgments of postural misuse, some pioneering work has been initiated to develop scales for more standardized measurement of muscle misuses associated with speech and voice disorders (Harris & Lieberman, 1993; Lieberman, 1994; Morrison & Rammage, 1993; Morrison & Rammage, with: Nichol, Pullan, May, & Salkeld, 1994; Morrison, Rammage, Belisle, Pullan, & Nichol, 1983). Electromyography may be used, in some instances, to measure muscle activity levels associated with postural misuses.

Electromyography: Three electrodiagnostic approaches—electromyography, neuromyography, and reflexmyography—are currently available for studying the electrical activity of laryngeal muscles. Of these methods, only electromyography (EMG) permits objective measurement of a muscle's activity (Thumfart, 1988). Because of its ability to aid in the assessment of a wide range of vocal abnormalities, including the muscle misuse dysphonias, and to generate objective, clinical data, EMG has become a valuable diagnostic tool, used routinely in some voice specialty clinics. The procedure is particularly useful in several specific types of cases: in distinguishing arytenoid fixation from vocal fold paralysis in patients who have suffered traumatic injuries to the larynx; when planning treatment for laryngeal paralysis depends on determining if there are signs of reinnervation activity; and in documenting the presence of laryngeal tremor or spasmodic activity in patients with suspected laryngeal dystonias.

Advances in Assessment Methodologies

As a clinical field matures it becomes account-able in large part through the specifications of its methods, both for the purpose of consistent application and for the purpose of demonstrated accomplishment. Unless and until a clinical field can specify its methods, the knowledge of that field cannot be scientifically validated. (Yoder, 1988)

Until recently, the field of voice disorders has lacked both assessment tools and consistent methodologies. Today, as a result of the greater availability of diagnostic instruments, voice assessment methodologies are gradually becoming more defined and systematic.

Although much remains to be accomplished with respect to standardization in voice assessment, some basic procedural processes can now be conceptualized (Figure 1–1). The contemporary model of the assessment process is premised on the development of a clinical hypothesis that can be either accepted or rejected through clinical observations and instrumental testing. A series of logical steps—case history interview, observational assessment, instrumental evaluation, and interdisciplinary referral—embody the clinical decision-making process.

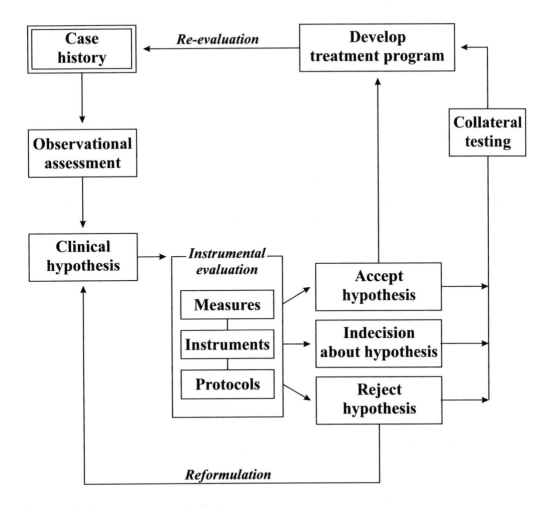

Figure I–I. Contemporary model of voice assessment.

Developing a Clinical Hypothesis

Voice assessment begins with a case history interview and observational assessment. (These topics are detailed in Chapters 2 and 3.) On the basis of the patient's history and the presenting signs and symptoms, clinicians formulate a clinical hypothesis that explains the voice problem. For example, if a patient reports multiple symptoms of gastroesophageal reflux (e.g., frequent heartburn, night coughing and choking, bitter taste in the morning) and accompanying voice and laryngeal symptoms (e.g., vocal fatigue, pain radiating toward one ear), reflux laryngitis or a contact ulcer might be suspected. Or, if an older patient complains of an inexplicably weak and breathy voice quality that has gradually worsened over the past 5 to 10 years, voice changes related to aging (presby-laryngis) or to a progressive neurological disorder might be considered as possible causes. In either scenario, decisions about how to proceed with further diagnostic testing are influenced by the clinical hypothesis that will be proved or disproved through observational and instrumental analysis.

Delineating Needed Measures

Depending on the clinical hypothesis, various subsets of instrumental examinations and protocols may be selected to yield essential test measures. Of all the instrumental measures of voice that can be used as part of a comprehensive evaluation, some are obtained routinely on all voice patients (e.g., laryngeal mirror images) and others might be indicated by the specific nature of the voice problem (e.g., electromyography).

Example of Measurement Delineation

Case history: A 66-year-old male with a prior history of glottic cancer ($T_1N_0M_0$) had received radiation therapy treatments 10 months previously. Following this treatment, there had been no recurrence of cancer. The presenting complaint was hoarseness that commenced shortly after the start of his radiation therapy treatments.

Observational assessment: Perceptually, his speaking voice was judged to be moderately harsh and breathy, with a reduced loudness level and elevated pitch. No other significant auditory or visual characteristics were evident.

Clinical hypothesis: On the basis of the patient's history and the perceptual characteristics of his speaking voice, it was hypothesized that the dysphonia was a sequela of radiation therapy, with characteristic changes in stiffness and mass, and compensatory muscle misuse. Although cancer recurrence was not suspected, further vocal function testing was needed to rule out this possiblity.

Instrumental evaluation: In addition to the physical examination that included indirect laryngoscopy (examination of the larynx by observing reflected images of the larynx in a laryneal mirror), the following instrumental measures were needed for voice assessment:

▶ Measures of VOCAL FOLD VIBRATION, since changes in the stiffness and mass of the vocal folds can result from radiation therapy and affect the vibratory patterns of the vocal folds during phonation (Lehman, Bless, & Brandenburg, 1988).
▶ Measures of the ACOUSTICS OF VOICE, since changes in stiffness and mass may alter fundamental frequency, intensity, and other acoustic parameters such as jitter, shimmer, and signal-to-noise ratio (Hirano & Bless, 1993).
▶ Measures of AERODYNAMIC FUNCTIONING, since compensatory muscle misuse and irregular glottic closure (potential complications of radiation therapy) can change the phonation threshold pressures and flows associated with voice production.

These measures and others are expanded upon in Chapter 4.

Confirming or Denying the Hypothesis

Following measurement selection and subsequent procedure/protocol selection, clinicians are in a position to either accept or reject their clinical hypothesis. Acceptance may lead directly to the development of a treatment plan; rejection necessitates reformulation and regeneration of an alternate hypothesis. In either instance—or when indecision prevails—additional, collateral information (e.g., MRI, CT, EMG, videofluoroscopy, allergy testing, endocrinology work-up, biopsy, or psychiatric evaluation) may be necessary for differential diagnosis or treatment planning.

Advances in Treatment Approaches and Procedures

New management approaches, designed to treat laryngeal disorders through surgical/medical or behavioral intervention (or both), have made treatment programs increasingly effective. Access to a wider range of tools and techniques has contributed to these advancements.

Surgical/Medical Management

A number of technological and procedural innovations demonstrate the progress that has been realized in surgical and medical aspects of voice care. Major innovations include microsurgery, radiation therapy, and the use of injectable substances.

Microsurgery: Advances in the 1960s culminated in the introduction of dissection of minute laryngeal structures under the microscope, with extremely fine instruments. As a result, the primary aim of laryngeal surgery shifted from removing disease to restoring voice (Ford & Bless, 1991). Today, phonosurgery improves or restores the voices of patients with benign vocal fold lesions (e.g., polyps, cysts, and granulomas), structurally impaired vocal folds (e.g., webs, scars, and sulci vocalis), and those whose vocal fold structure is intact but is incapable of movement (e.g., unilateral vocal fold paralysis).

In addition to better preserving the voice, laryngologists now have access to a wider range of surgical interventions. In treating patients with unilateral vocal fold paralysis, for example, at least four surgical possibilities exist in addition to the vocal fold injection techniques. They include the thyroplasty type I medialization procedure (Isshiki, Okamura, & Ishikawa, 1975; Koufman, 1986), an arytenoid adduction (Koufman, 1991), laryngeal reinnervation surgery (Crumley, 1991), and a combination of these procedures.

Laryngeal conservation surgeries developed to eradicate cancer without total removal of the larynx have become more viable treatment options for many because of earlier detection and diagnosis of the disease. The laser cordectomy (Hirano, Hirade, & Kawasaki, 1985), the near-total laryngectomy (Pearson, 1985), and the standard hemilaryngectomy (Biller, Ogura, & Pratt, 1971) are three prime examples of laryngeal conservation surgeries.

In cases where a complete laryngectomy is necessary, innovative techniques such as the tracheoesophageal puncture (TEP) developed by Singer and Blom (1980) and the neoglottic technique of laryngeal conservation (Brandenburg, 1980; Brandenburg, Cragle, & Rammage, 1991) allow patients to speak again through use of either a prosthetic device or a surgically created shunt, respectively.

Radiation Therapy: An alternative to surgery is the use of radiation therapy (XRT) or, in some cases, combined surgery and XRT. Advances in computer technology and more exact methods of delivery such as use of sophisticated linear accelerators now allow radiation oncologists to target cancer cells more precisely and to better protect normal cells from the toxic effects of radiation (Pellitteri, Kennedy, Vrabec, Beiler, & Hellstrom, 1991).

Injectable Substances: The emergence of new injectable substances for adding mass to the vocal folds has vastly improved the effectiveness of treating glottic incompetence. Injectable substances now used in the United States to permanently augment paralyzed vocal folds include polytetrafluoroethylene (Teflon®) (Arnold, 1962; Fried, 1988), autogenous fat (Brandenburg, Kirkham, & Koschkee, 1992), and autologous collagen (Ford, personal communication, 1994). In some clinics, silicon (Hirano, Tanaka, & Hibi, 1990) and bovine collagen (Ford & Bless, 1993) are also used for this purpose.

Another injectable substance, botulinum toxin, has become the most commonly used treatment for spasmodic dysphonia (SD). Its effectiveness in relieving spasms of the larynx has been well documented (Blitzer & Brin, 1992; Ludlow, 1990). In general, these investigators have demonstrated that injections of botulinum toxin into selected muscles of the larynx can produce a temporary paralysis or muscle weakness, generally lasting from 3 to 6 months, that alleviates muscle spasms and improves the voices of many patients with SD.

Behavioral Management

Within the domain of behavioral intervention for vocal pathologies, recent advances have increased both the objectivity and the effectiveness of clinical treatment programs. Three fundamental changes have greatly influenced behavioral management programming: improved quantification methods, physiological voice therapy, and the increased availability of behavioral treatments.

Quantification: Before technology was introduced into the clinic, it was generally acknowledged that behavioral voice therapy could improve some patients' voices. Only rudimentary tools, however, were available for documenting change. Typically, improvements in voice were based on patients' reports (e.g., "feeling less vocal fatigue") or clinicians' observations (e.g., "the voice sounds clearer and stronger"). In other words, perceptual judgments and sensory symptoms were the primary basis for determining if

change had occurred. With the integration of sophisticated technologies into clinical practice, the effectiveness of behavioral treatments is no longer questionable. Speech pathologists can now objectively quantify the effects of their voice therapies by establishing baseline stability prior to treatment, monitoring the course of change, and documenting the outcomes of treatment using tests of vocal function described above and in Chapter 4. Suggested formats for baselining and monitoring progress are discussed in Chapter 6.

Physiological Voice Therapy: A second important development in behavioral management relates to the speech pathologist's ability to approach voice therapy from a physiological viewpoint rather than from a purely auditory-perceptual or symptomatic perspective. Physiological voice therapy is distinct from symptomatic voice therapy. Symptomatic therapy focuses on the modification of deviant vocal symptoms such as breathiness, low pitch, and hard glottal attacks as a means for improving voice quality (Stemple, 1993). In contrast, physiological voice therapy is a behavioral treatment approach directed toward the modification of a patient's phonatory physiology or laryngeal functioning (e.g., improved glottic closure, increased mean airflow rate, or decreased vocal intensity). As a sequela to physiological voice therapy, morphologic and structural changes can ensue (e.g., elimination of vocal nodules, reduction of Reinke's edema, decreased vocal fold inflammation).

Of course, to develop measurable, physiologically based treatment objectives, clinicians must have access to appropriate equipment and instrumentation. They must also be knowledgeable about normative data for various age groups—children, adolescents, young and middle-aged adults, and geriatric individuals—and have a current understanding of both normal and abnormal anatomy and phonatory physiology.

Example of Physiologically Based Goals

Case history: A 78-year-old male patient came to the Voice Clinic complaining of a weak and breathy speaking voice that had gradually worsened over the previous 5 years.

Observational assessment: Perceptually, his speaking voice was characterized by an asthenic (weak) and breathy quality, monotone intonation pattern, and a reduced loudness level. His phrases were short, generally four to five words in length.

Clinical hypothesis: It was hypothesized that the patient's voice problems were hypofunctional in nature and likely related primarily to the aging process.

Instrumental evaluation: Indirect mirror examination did not reveal any organic laryngeal pathology, but glottal incompetence was evident. During videostroboscopic evaluation, a glottal gap, extending along the entire length of the vocal folds, was visualized along with bilateral vocal fold bowing and an absent closed phase to the vibratory cycle. Aerodynamic and acoustic testing demonstrated low mean airflow rates (35 cc/sec), low phonation threshold pressures (2 cm H_2O), low conversational intensity (54 dB) compared to normative data for his age and gender, and low conversational fundamental frequency (f_0) mean (100 Hz) compared to his spontaneous vocalizations (e.g., laughter, "umhum" at 165 Hz). Stimulability testing using videoendoscopy revealed better closure during a cough and other effort closure activities. However, these activities also created hyperadduction in the patient's supraglottal structures. Additional probe testing explored closure during humming exercises and coordinated voice onsets: both were associated with better glottic closure without hyperadduction in supraglottic structures, and both were produced in an f_0 range deemed more appropriate for the patient's age and gender.

Acceptance of the hypothesis: All of these instrumental findings were consistent with the respiratory and phonatory patterns commonly exhibited by geriatric patients, with hypoadduction voice problems related to aging, and with a tendency to maintain an inappropriately low speaking pitch. Therefore, the clinical hypothesis was accepted. A pretreatment vocal function profile was generated and voice therapy was recommended.

Treatment planning: Prior to initiating exercises for respiratory and laryngeal muscle strengthening, five physiologically based therapy goals were established:

▶ obtain complete glottic closure during posttreatment videostroboscopic examination,
▶ obtain mean airflow rates of 80 cc/sec or more during sustained vowel productions,
▶ obtain phonation threshold pressures of at least 4 cm H_2O during repetitions of the syllable /pi/,
▶ obtain intensity levels of 70 dB or greater during conversational speech, and
▶ maintain a mean conversational f_0 of 150 Hz or higher.

Availability of Behavioral Treatments: An expanded repertoire of behavioral treatments has become available to the speech pathologist managing voice disorders. Clinicians now have access to traditional methodologies (e.g., vocal hygiene counseling, relaxation therapies, and resonance exercises) as well as more contemporary treatment approaches. Newer treatment approaches range from instrumental biofeedback to holistic (whole-system) techniques such as the Accent Method (Kotby, 1994) and the Laryngeal

Muscle Strengthening Exercises Program (Stemple, 1993) to the manual laryngeal musculoskeletal tension reduction technique (Aronson, 1990; Roy & Leeper, 1993).

One procedure that has proven to be particularly beneficial in both therapy planning and implementation is a visual feedback technique using videoendoscopy—an endoscope, either rigid transoral or flexible transnasal, connected to a video system, to allow imaging of the larynx. The patient phonates using a variety of stimulability or probe therapy techniques while the patient and clinicians observe accompanying changes in laryngeal function. This approach can aid in treatment planning or be implemented as a visual feedback method. Since the technique provides real-time visual feedback to patients about both breathing and phonatory patterns within the larynx, it has become a highly valued approach for treating patients with paradoxical vocal cord dysfunction, a breathing disorder characterized by adduction of the true vocal cords on inspiration and abduction on expiration. The technique can also offer useful information to physicians considering vocal fold medialization. Manual compression tasks (e.g., manually compressing the thryoid alae) can be performed using endoscopy to preview the likely effects of medialization. A more detailed discussion of probe therapy using videoendoscopy follows in Chapter 6.

Changes in Professional Roles and Relationships

The traditional medical model of service delivery has also undergone fundamental changes. While the roles of the laryngologist and speech pathologist remain central to voice care delivery, other specialists such as singing and/or drama teachers, physical therapists, psychiatrists and psychologists, neurologists, and other medical specialists now play greater roles than previously. Because voice patients often require more than a medical evaluation, an increasing trend toward interdisciplinary care has evolved in many voice specialty clinics. Although various models of team functioning can be found in different medical centers, the objective of the interdisciplinary team approach remains the same—to provide a higher quality of care to patients through the collaborative efforts of experts in different specialties.

The Voice Care Team

The composition of the voice care team may change from one patient to another, depending on the potential diagnosis and each individual's needs. For example, in the evaluation of a patient with suspected paradoxical vocal cord dysfunction, input from the allergist, the pulmonologist, the speech pathologist, the laryngologist, and the psychiatrist might all be required for differential diagnosis. For a professional voice user, team members might include the laryngologist, the speech pathologist, and the singing specialist.

Only two team members—the laryngologist and the speech pathologist—are routinely involved in the assessment of all voice patients. Depending on the physical setting, the patient population, available financial and technical resources, and individual personalities, the interface between these professionals can vary; yet their ongoing collaboration has become vital to the success of any diagnostic or treatment program.

In their collaboration for voice-disordered patients, the laryngologist and the speech pathologist provide services that naturally complement one another. Whereas the laryngologist diagnoses diseases of the larynx, the speech pathologist evaluates vocal disorders resulting from laryngeal disease. Whereas the laryngologist performs a physical examination of the larynx, the speech pathologist examines the physiological manifestations of laryngeal function. Whereas the laryngologist manages voice problems by prescribing medications and/or performing surgery, the speech pathologist intervenes by conducting behavioral voice therapy. Cooperative efforts involving the expertise of both professionals are becoming increasingly prevalent both in and out of the clinical environment. In the clinic, approaches such as probe therapy utilizing videoendoscopy are being used regularly by some laryngology/speech pathology teams. Although the speech pathologist generally conducts this type of stimulability testing at the end of a videostroboscopic evaluation, both the speech pathologist and laryngologist might assess the auditory perceptual and physiological changes that occur when probe therapy is conducted cooperatively.

During intraoperative monitoring, the laryngologist and speech pathologist may work as partners in the operating room, as, for example, during the Isshiki Type I thyroplasty. The speech pathologist may assist the surgeon by visually and auditorily monitoring the patient, who is asked to phonate as a silastic implant is surgically introduced. Through collaborative efforts such as this, optimal phonosurgical results are obtained.

Collaboration with other professionals is a commonly accepted practice in the modern clinical voice laboratory. The frequent participation of singing or drama pedagogues in assessing and managing professional voice users is one example. The speech pathologist and voice pedagogue may collaborate on behalf of a patient to ensure that the goals and techniques introduced by the two voice care professionals are compatible for both speaking and vocal performance activities. Similarly, the speech pathologist may collaborate with the psychiatrist on behalf of a patient with a psychogenic dysphonia to ensure that common assumptions, goals, and techniques are reinforced by the two professionals.

Changes in Cost of Services

The 1970s and 1980s were times of rapid technological advancement, but they also marked the beginning of unparalleled growth in health care expenditures. Primary factors that have contributed to these increases include high-technology instrumentation, increased specialization, and competitive marketing in the health care industry. These advances have not come without some investments—and therefore costs—for all involved in voice care. Changes in costs make it imperative that voice care today be as efficient and effective as possible.

Costs to Patients

In recent years, patients have been subjected to a continual rise in fees for service. Fee increases have, at least in part, been attributable to the increased costs associated with high-technology examinations. In addition, many nonmonetary costs accrue to patients, including invasiveness of procedures, risks associated with examinations and treatments, time spent undergoing comprehensive diagnostic testing, possible post-treatment deficits or complications, and recovery time following intervention. Although the overall benefits of services generally outweigh the disadvantages, the impact of these financial and personal costs to consumers should not be minimized.

Costs to Practitioners

Health care professionals involved in the diagnosis and treatment of voice problems in the 1990s are facing many new challenges. The evolving technologies that bring opportunities for learning and professional growth also place greater demands on all members of the health care team. For example, to meet state-of-the-art standards, professionals must regularly examine their beliefs, procedures, and instrumentation and replace those that are obsolete. Financially, this means generating increased revenues to cover the costs of new equipment. Educationally, this means seeking opportunities for continuing education, to remain professionally current. A second challenge faced by today's health care professionals is that of maintaining quality human interactions in an age of increasing technology. The arts of observation and interview continue to be critical to differential diagnosis. Yet, as more time is spent administering impersonal, instrumental tests, less time is available to explore the psychological and social aspects of voice and communication. Consequently, practitioners must exercise their observation and interview skills throughout the course of the evaluation to remain cost-effective while being responsive to the patient's emotional needs. They must also have well-established criteria for referral to other specialities—such as psychiatry—so that appropriate recommendations can be made when needed.

Costs to Institutions

The yearly costs to institutions for equipment have skyrocketed with the purchase of new high-technology tools. Consider, for example, the costs incurred by institutions for MRI in 1994: purchase prices alone ranged from 1.5 to 3 *million* dollars. Costs of physical space, salaries, supplies, patient accommodations, and the marketing of services have also risen relentlessly. These costs are passed on to the patient or health insurer. The resulting system feeds into itself (Figure 1–2). Yet, every patient whose quality of life has been improved or restored by these technological advances would testify to their worth, for the ultimate goal continues to be the benefit to the patient (Table 1–1).

GOALS OF VOICE CARE IN THE MEDICAL SETTING

Clinical expertise, research, and technology have combined in the medical setting to pro-vide voice patients and their families with a higher standard of voice care (Table 1–2). Future benefits to patients and the medical community will be realized by continuing efforts to streamline diagnostic procedures, develop greater standardization in clinical examinations of voice, to educate each other about our fields of specialty, and engage in innovative clinical research. The chapters that follow discuss these current and future directions in voice care, beginning with a full assessment of the patients' conditions and needs.

REFERENCES

Arnold, G. E. (1962). Vocal rehabilitation of paralytic dysphonia. *Archives of Otolaryngology, 76,* 358.

Aronson, A. E. (1990). *Clinical voice disorders* (3rd ed.). New York: Thieme Stratton.

Biller, H. F., Ogura, J. H., & Pratt, L. L. (1971). Hemilaryngectomy for T2 glottic cancers. *Archives of Otolaryngology, 93,* 238–243.

Bless, D. M., Hirano, M., & Feder, R. J. (1987). Videostroboscopic evaluation of the larynx. *Ear, Nose and Throat Journal, 66*(7), 289–296.

Blitzer, A., & Brin. M. F. (1992). Treatment of spasmodic dysphonia (laryngeal dystonia) with local injections of botulinum toxin. *Journal of Voice, 6*(4), 356–369.

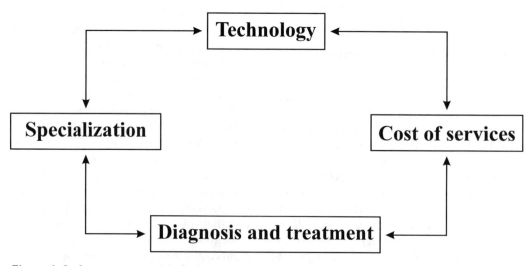

Figure 1–2. Servo-system model of voice care.

TABLE 1–1. Recent changes in patient services.

	Medical Technology	*Clinical Practice*
Diagnostic techniques	► MRI ► CT ► Ultrasonography ► Videofluoroscopy ► Videostroboscopy ► Analysis of vocal function ► EMG	► Laryngeal imaging ► Instrumental and noninstrumental protocols ► Diagnostic probe therapy
Assessment methodologies	► Objective instrumental tools	► Contemporary assessment models
Treatment procedures	► Microsurgical tools ► X-ray linear accelerators ► Injectable substances ► Visual feedback devices ► Augmentative aids and systems (e.g., voice amplifiers)	► Microsurgical techniques ► Methods for delivering radiation therapy ► Injection methods ► Behavioral therapy techniques
Professional roles	► Specialization ► Technological expertise ► Clinical laboratory development ► Continuing education	► Interdisciplinary collaboration ► Marketing services ► Quality assurance ► Program development ► Staff education
Patient costs	► Higher fees ► Time ► Invasiveness of procedures ► Risks/Complications	► Less human interaction ► Lengthy history questionnaires ► Multiple clinic visits
Patient benefits	► Objective, instrumental voice analysis ► Precise treatment planning and monitoring ► Expanded treatment options ► Patient and family education	► Specialty clinics ► Comprehensive/coordinated care ► Combination modality treatments

13

TABLE 1–2. Contemporary voice care programs offer.

In-depth case history interviews

Informal, observational assessments

Instrumental analyses

Interdisciplinary collaboration

Differential diagnosis of psychogenic, neurogenic, systemic, and behavioral problems

Voice screenings

Preventative counseling

Early detection of life-threatening conditions

Precise treatment planning and monitoring

Treatments for previously untreatable conditions

Combination modality treatments

Less invasive procedures

Shortened hospital stays

Reduced recovery periods

Pre- and postoperative counseling

Individual and group therapy programs

Assistive and augmentative device training

Support groups

Home-programming

Bohme, G. (1989) Clinical contribution to ultrasound diagnosis of the larynx (German). *Laryngo-Rhino-Otologie, 68*(9), 510–515.

Brandenburg, J. H. (1980) Vocal rehabilitation after laryngectomy. *Archives of Otolaryngology, 106,* 688–691.

Brandenburg, J. H., Cragle, S. P,. & Rammage, L. A. (1991). A modified neoglottis procedure: Update and analysis. *Otolaryngology—Head and Neck Surgery, 104*(2), 175–181.

Brandenburg, J. H., Kirkham, W. R., & Koschkee, D. C. (1992). Vocal cord augmentation with autogenous fat. *Laryngoscope, 102,* 495–500.

Colton, R. H., & Casper, J. K. (1990). *Understanding voice problems: A physiological perspective for diagnosis and treatment.* Baltimore: Williams & Wilkins.

Crumley, R. L. (1991). *Laryngeal reinnervation techniques in phonosurgery: Assessment and surgical management of voice disorders.* New York: Raven Press.

Edberg, O. (1992). Radiologic evaluation of swallowing. In M. E. Groher (Ed.), *Dysphagia diagnosis and management* (2nd ed.). Boston: Butterworth-Heinemann.

Ford, C. N., & Bless, D. M. (1991). *Phonosurgery: Assessment and surgical management of voice disorders.* New York: Raven Press.

Ford, C. N., & Bless, D. B. (1993). Selected problems treated by vocal fold injection of collagen. *American Journal of Otolaryngology, 14*(4), 257–261.

Fried, M. P. (1988). *The larynx: A multidisciplinary approach.* Boston: Little, Brown.

Harris, T., & Lieberman, J. (1993). The cricothyroid mechanism, its relation to vocal fatigue and vocal dysfunction. *Voice, 2,* 89–96.

Hirano, M., & Bless, D. M. (1993). *Videostroboscopic examination of the larynx.* San Diego: Singular Publishing Group.

Hirano, M., Hirade, Y., & Kawasaki, H. (1985). Vocal function following carbon dioxide laser surgery for glottic carcinoma. *Annals of Otology, Rhinology and Laryngology, 94,* 232–235.

Hirano, M., Tanaka, S., & Hibi, S. (1990). Transcutaneous intrafold injection for unilateral vocal fold paralysis: Functional results. *Annals of Otology, Rhinology and Laryngology, 99*(8), 598–604.

Isshiki, N., Okamura, H., & Ishikawa, T. (1975). Thyroplasty Type I (Iateral compression) for dysphonia due to vocal cord paralysis or atrophy. *Acta Otololaryngologica (Stockholm), 80,* 465–473.

Kotby, M. N. (1994). *The accent method of voice therapy.* San Diego: Singular Publishing Group.

Koufman, J. A. (1986). Laryngoplasty for vocal cord medialization: An alternative to Teflon. *Laryngoscope, 96,* 726.

Koufman, J. A. (1991, May). *Medialization laryngoplasty and the arytenoid adduction procedure: Which and when?* Paper presented at the Annual Meeting of the American Otolaryngological Association, Waikoloa, HI.

Kuhns, L. R., Thornburg, J. R., & Fryback, D. G. (1989). *Decision making in imaging.* Chicago: Year Book Medical Publications.

Laver, J., & MacKenzie-Beck, J. (1991). *Vocal profile analysis.* Edinburgh: University of Edinburgh, Queen Margaret College.

Lehman, J. J., Bless, D. M., & Brandenburg, J. H. (1988). An objective assessment of voice production after radiation therapy for Stage I squamous cell carcinoma of the glottis. *Otolaryngology—Head and Neck Surgery, 98,* 121–129.

Lieberman, J. (1994). *Lieberman postural assessment for hyperfunctional dysphonia.* Sidcup, Kent: Queen Mary's Hospital Voice Disorder Research Laboratory.

Ludlow. C. L. (1990). Treatment of speech and voice disorders with botulinum toxin. *Journal of American Medical Association, 264,* 2671–2675.

Mafee, M. F., Langer, B., Valvassori, G., Soboroff, B. J., & Friedman, M. (1986). Radiologic diagnosis of nonsquamous tumors of the head and neck. *Otolaryngologic Clinics of North America, 19*(3).

McWilliams, B. J., Morris, H. L., & Shelton, R. L. (1990). *Cleft palate speech* (2nd ed.). Philadelphia: B.C. Decker.

Morrison, M. D., & Rammage, L. A. (1993). Muscle misuse voice disorders: Description and classification. *Acta Otolaryngologica, 113,* 428–434

Morrison, M. D., Rammage, L. A., Belisle, G., Pullan, B., & Nichol, H. (1983). Muscular tension dysphonia. *Journal of Otolaryngology, 12,* 302–306.

Morrison, M., & Rammage, L., with: Nichol, H., Pullan, B., May, P., & Salkeld, L. (1994). *The management of voice disorders.* London: Chapman & Hall, Medical.

Pearson, B. W. (1985). The theory and technique of near-total laryngectomy. In B. J. Biller & H. F. Biller (Eds.), *Surgery of the larynx.* Philadelphia: W. B. Saunders.

Pellitteri, P. K., Kennedy, T. L., Vrabec, D. P., Beiler, D., & Hellstrom, M. (1991). Radiotherapy. The mainstay in the treatment of early glottic carcinoma. *Archives of Otolaryngology—Head and Neck Surgery, 117,* 297–301.

Roy, N., & Leeper, H. A. (1993). Effects of manual laryngeal musculoskeletal tension reduction technique as a treatment for functional voice disorders; Perceptual and acoustic measures, *Journal of Voice, 7*(3), 242–249.

Schaeffer, S. D. (1991). Use of CT scanning in the management of the acutely injured larynx. *Otolaryngologic Clinics of North America: Current Issues of Head and Neck Trauma, 24*(1).

Singer, M. I., & Blom, E. D. (1980). An endoscopic technique for restoration of voice after laryngectomy. *Annals of Otology, Rhinology and Laryngology, 89,* 529–533.

Sloane, P. M., Griffin, J. M., & O'Dwyer, T. P. (1991). Esophageal insufflation and videofluoroscopy for evaluation of esophageal speech in laryngectomy patients: Clinical implications. *Radiology, 181,* 433–437.

Stemple, J. C. (1993). *Voice therapy clinical studies.* St. Louis: Mosby-Year Book.

Thumfart, W. F. (1988). Electrodialysis of laryngeal nerve disorders. *Ear, Nose and Throat Journal, 67,* 380–393.

Unger, J. (1987). *Head and neck imaging.* New York: Churchill Livingstone.

Woo, P., Colton, R., Casper, J., & Brewer, D. (1991). Diagnostic value of stroboscopic examination in hoarse patients. *Journal of Voice, 5*(3), 231–238.

Yoder, D. E., & Kent, R. D. (1988). *Decision making in speech-language pathology.* Philadelphia: B. C. Decker.

CHAPTER

THE PATIENT HISTORY

The Science of the Diagnostic Interview

Against a background of science and technology, real-life human dramas unfold through the process of voice assessment. The scripts detail information about patients—details that can alter assessment methods, influence diagnoses, and determine prognoses and therapeutic outcomes. The personal interview is the scene in which clinicians define many of these assessment and treatment variables, using the techniques of diagnostic interview and observational assessment.

During the personal interview, clinicians elicit relevant case history information and identify related medical, psychological, and behavioral problems. Together, these components, *the diagnostic interview* and *observational assessment*, form the complete patient history. Because the history offers critical information to the evaluation process and is essential to clinical hypothesis development, these topics are discussed in detail here. This chapter focuses on the science of the diagnostic interview; Chapter 3 describes the art of observational assessment.

THE DIAGNOSTIC INTERVIEW

The science (of the diagnostic interview) is the knowledge base that guides the selection of questions and informs the interpretation of responses. (Colton & Casper, 1990, p. 165).

Two assessment instruments, the history questionnaire and the personal interview, are used to obtain in-depth case history information. The clinical expertise required to use these diagnostic tools effectively and to interpret their significance should not be underestimated. In actual clinical practice, novice clinicians generally master the technical skills needed to perform "high technology" laboratory tests and examinations long before they acquire the knowledge and skills needed to conduct proficient case history interviews. Perhaps this pattern of learning is a product of the unpredictable nature of human interactions.

Patients bring to the clinical setting different sets of problems, motivations, and expectations. Some patients are extremely receptive and cooperative during the initial interview; others react with hostility and anger. Some are overly verbal; others hesitate to express their feelings and concerns. Some deny their own habits such as alcoholism or drug abuse; others dramatically amplify their problems. Some patients seek autonomy in decision making; others demonstrate dependency. Experience combined with knowledge enables the voice clinician to recognize and resonate to these differing perspectives, and educe essential case history information by responding to specific patients' needs.

Throughout the interview process, the patient needs to assume several responsibilities. One responsibility is to provide accurate and detailed accounts of past and present circumstances that might influence vocal functioning. Openness and honesty in reporting personal information is essential if an accurate diagnosis is to be reached. Questions about personal habits, behaviors, and feelings are routinely posed in conjunction with the standard voice history. In some situations, sensitive personal information must be elicited with direct questioning, either on a written history questionnaire or verbally:

"During the past year, have you had any problems with drinking? Smoking? Drugs? Dieting? Sleeping? Fatigue?"

"Are you presently using birth control pills? Fertility drugs? Hormonal supplements?"

"Do you have any sexually transmitted health problems such as herpes? Syphillis? Gonorrhea? HIV virus?"

"Have there been any major problems at home with your spouse? Partner? Boyfriend? Girlfriend? Parents? Children? Finances?"

"Have you found yourself recently being short-tempered? Easily upset? Crying frequently?"

"Do you tend to internalize anger rather than expressing it verbally?"

"Have you ever consulted a psychologist or psychiatrist? if so, why?"

Of course, the diagnostic interview should not become an interrogation. Nevertheless, these examples illustrate the highly personal nature of the medical voice history and underscore the necessity for strict patient confidentiality. They also touch on two other issues: the importance of wording questions in an inoffensive, professional manner and the need to provide at least a general rationale for questions that might appear unrelated to the voice problem. If clinicians do not offer basic rationales for questions, the patient's "goodwill" is often sacrificed and resistance can develop. Together the patient and the voice-team diagnosticians determine the course of the diagnostic interview. The script they create collectively will define professional relationships that extend beyond the interview itself.

History Questionnaires

In general, written documentation serves as the clinician's entry point into the patient's life and problems. For an inpatient in an acute care setting, practitioners usually rely on the collection of history forms, dictated reports, and clinical notes found in the hospital chart. These patients are generally quite ill and their energies are best spent on the clinical examination.

In contrast, outpatients being seen for an initial visit may receive lengthy questionnaires. Many specialty clinics mail patients comprehensive history forms to be completed prior to the evaluation. This "survey method" of case history collection was developed in medical settings during the 1950s in response to proclamations by social scientists that interview by questionnaire is a valid and time-efficient tool for taking a history (Billings & Stoeckle, 1989).

Over the years, the formats and methods of administration have been revolutionized, but the basic principles remain unaltered. Questionnaires enhance data collection by ensuring consistent, systematic, and comprehensive methodology; consolidating pertinent background information into an abbreviated, manageable form; identifying key areas of inquiry prior to the personal interview; freeing clinicians from tedious, nonpatient-centered activities such as note-taking; and saving health care professionals' time.

Recent evolutionary approaches to the history collection process have included computer-administered questionnaires (Coulehan & Block, 1992), the use of telecommunication devices (Castle, 1982), and speech synthesis systems (e.g., Laver & MacKenzie-Beck, 1992). In the first instance, patients put biographical data directly into a computer that generates a printout of the case history information. In the second case, telecommunication systems such as the Telecommunication Device for the Deaf (TDD) enable hearing-impaired, speech-impaired, or voice-impaired individuals to communicate and respond through the telephone system via portable, typewriter-style units. More recently, advances in speech technology have brought sophisticated speech synthesis systems that allow patients to interact with a machine capable of asking questions and responding to a fairly wide range of patient responses and queries. Although current use of speech synthesis systems is limited because of prohibitive costs, this technology will soon play a significant role in enhancing voice care programs.

Regardless of the collection method, the information obtained from the written history provides the clinician with a microcosmic view of the patient's history, behaviors, lifestyle, stressors, and voice usage. The information also directs the health care professional toward areas of concern that can be more thoroughly explored in the personal interview. Additionally, the patient's perspective of the problem can be determined, using self-evaluation questionnaires, such as the Voice Disability Index (Appendix 2–1) (Koschkee, 1993).

Because different populations present different sets of problems, the use of specialized questionnaires can facilitate the diagnostic interview process. Specialized history forms have been developed for pediatrics professional voice users (Appendix 2–2, Sataloff, 1991), and patients with paradoxical vocal cord dysfunction (Appendix 2–3, Bless, 1994); spasmodic dysphonias (Appendix 2–4, Bless & Ford, 1989); and unilateral vocal fold paralysis (Appendix 2–5). In the discussion that follows, the focus is broader in its scope: history-taking in children and adults.

The Pediatric History

During the evaluation of children, it is important to know the history of the voice problem as well as the general developmental history, medical history, familial history, voice usage, and family and social interaction patterns (Table 2–1). This type of comprehensive background information provides clues to the etiology of the voice disorder that can be subsequently confirmed or denied through clinical testing and examination.

Pediatric questionnaire development and interpretation require a thorough knowledge of normal development and the voice disorders commonly experienced by children at various maturational stages. The problems presented by the newborn (birth to 9 weeks), the infant (9 weeks to 18 months), the toddler (18 months to 3 years), the preschooler (3 to 6 years), the child (6 to 12 years), and the adolescent (12 to 17 years) may be distinct: anatomically, endocrinologically, psychologically, and behaviorally. Consequently, the etiologic bases of their voice disorders may differ. For example, voice problems in a newborn likely relate to a congenital anomaly or birth defect, a genetic disorder, or an iatrogenic injury suffered during labor, delivery, or the neonatal period. In contrast, the majority of

TABLE 2–1. Elements of the pediatric voice history.

Voice history	▸ Past and present symptoms ▸ Onset and duration ▸ Clinical course and variability ▸ Previous evaluations and/or treatments
Medical history	▸ Major illnesses ▸ Surgeries ▸ Accidents and/or injuries ▸ Allergies ▸ Drug/medication use ▸ Relevant medical problems
Voice usage	▸ Excessive loudness ▸ Voice strain/tension ▸ Abusive habits ▸ Affective voice usage
Family history	▸ Familial diseases, illnesses, conditions ▸ Family dynamics, learning, environment
Developmental information	▸ Hearing history ▸ Gross- and fine-motor development ▸ Associated speech/language delays or disorders ▸ Cognitive development
Child's personal profile	▸ Personality ▸ Social interaction patterns ▸ Personal habits, behaviors, stresses

voice problems arising in a 3-year-old relate to respiratory illnesses, traumatic injuries to the larynx or airway, or associated developmental disorders or delays.

Age of onset alone cannot determine the nature of a child's problem, but it is one critical feature of the pediatric voice history. The general relationship between age as a predisposing factor and associated vocal pathologies is further delineated in Table 2–2. Other critical features of the pediatric voice history include symptomatology, clinical course, coexisting speech, language, or hearing problems, and the family's hereditary patterns.

Symptomatology: In children, as with adults, probes into symptomatology generally include questions about gastroesophageal reflux disease (GERD). GERD is a common but often neglected aspect of the pediatric voice history. Although reflux has

been linked to laryngeal disorders in adults (Batch, 1988; Earnest, 1991; Jones et al., 1990; Wilson et al., 1989), there is minimal recognition of the condition in children. Gray (1992), Contencin and Narcy (1992), and Olson (1991) have discussed the need to identify and manage GERD in the pediatric population. Whereas the diagnostic tests commonly used to diagnose reflux (e.g., 24-hour pH monitoring or upper gastrointestinal videofluoroscopic series) might not be well suited to children because of their invasive nature, symptoms of GERD can easily be explored during the history intake.

Does the child experience "classic" (GERD) symptoms such as dysphagia? Pain during swallowing (odynophagia)? Chronic coughing? Choking? Burping? Regurgitation? Vomiting?

Are there recurrent respiratory problems that might be related to "silent" refluxing such as

TABLE 2–2. Age as a factor in determining pediatric voice problems.

Age	High-risk Disorders/Conditions	Common Signs
Birth to 9 weeks	Congenital anomalies, birth defects, genetic disorders	Anterior laryngeal web, laryngomalacia, laryngeal cyst, cleft palate, hearing loss, Down syndrome, Cri-du-chat syndrome
	Injuries suffered during labor, delivery, or the neonatal period	Cerebral palsy, vocal fold paralysis, hemangioma
9 weeks to 18 mo.	Intubation injuries	Laryngeal swelling, infection, subglottic stenosis, posterior laryngeal web
18 mo. to 3 yrs.	Respiratory illnesses	Croup, respiratory obstruction, laryngeal swelling, reflux laryngitis
	Traumatic injuries to the airway/larynx	Laryngeal/airway injuries due to foreign body aspiration, ingestion of caustic agents, or intubation
	Related speech/language/hearing problems	Motor speech problems, language delays/disorders, hearing loss
3 to 6 yrs.	Inflammatory illnesses	Supraglottis (epiglottis)
	Hyperfunctional disorders	Vocal nodules
	Related speech and language problems	Fluency and voice problems
6 to 12 yrs.	Hyperfunctional disorders	Vocal nodules, polyps
	Viral infections	Juvenile papilloma
	Hereditary disorders manifested in childhood	Tourette syndrome, angioneurotic edema
12 to 17 yrs.	Anorexia/bulimia	Reflux laryngitis
	Exacerbation of asthmatic conditions	Paradoxical vocal fold disorders, exercise-induced asthma
	Changes related to puberty	Mutational falsetto (males)
	Hyperfunctional disorders	Vocal nodules, pseudocysts
	Traumatic injuries to the head and neck	Blunt or penetrating traumas from sport injuries, automobile accidents, or gunshot wounds

stridor? Recurrent croup? Obstructive apnea? Asthma? Paradoxical vocal cord motion? Recurrent pneumonia? Bronchitis?

Heartburn has not been included in the symptomatology here since it is not a commonly reported symptom in children as it is in adults (Burton, Pransky, Kearns, Katz, & Seid, 1992).

Respiratory distress is a common symptom of children suffering congenital laryn-geal diseases and primary organic lesions such as papillomatosis. Morrison, Rammage et al. (1994) distinguish between primary and secondary organic disorders in their description of common causes of voice and respiratory difficulties in children. For children who have hoarseness accompanied by symptoms such as respiratory distress, tachypnea, tachycardia, or cyanosis, it is important to determine if there is a related respiratory, circulatory, or cardiac condition (Heatley, 1992). In these cases, Heatley advocates a comprehensive work-up, including a thorough review of the child's medical history for evidence of recognized cardiac, neurological, or esophageal anomalies, as well as for information about the development of the problem (e.g., post-traumatic or postintubation onset).

Clinical Course: The clinical course of the problem is another key area for investigation.

Is the child's voice getting better, worse, or staying the same over time?

Does the voice deteriorate predictably during or following specific situations (e.g., yelling on the playground, crying before bedtime, fighting with siblings)?

Do seasonal variations suggest that allergies are a contributing factor?

Is the problem exacerbated when the child is tired or ill?

Does "worse" voice occur in the mornings when reflux problems or postnasal drip are most likely to influence voice?

Coexisting Communication Problems: Questions regarding hearing and speech and language development are important aspects of the child's general developmental history. Recent studies have demonstrated that combinations or clusters of communication disorders are common in children (Carlson, 1992). One recent study, involving a data base of nearly 39,000 school-age children, showed that voice problems co-existed with articulation disorders in more than 50% of the randomly sampled cases. Approximately 40% of the children with voice disorders exhibited reduced language performance, and those children with voice problems displayed significantly elevated hearing thresholds, when compared with the (normal voice) control group (St. Louis, Hansen, Buch, & Oliver, 1992). In a related study, St. Louis and Hinzman (1988) examined the coexistence of voice and stuttering problems. They found that two thirds of the children who stuttered also had voice deviancies. Coincidences of voice disorders and stuttering are further described by Baumgartner, Ramig, and Kuehn (1986). Shriberg, Kwiatkowski, Best, Hengst, and Terselic-Weber (1986) have reported on the incidence of voice disorders in children with general speech intelligibility problems. They found that over 50% of the 90 "speech-delayed" children in their study demonstrated some consistent voice differences in continuous speech, primarily in vocal quality. A high incidence of voice abnormalities, 84%, has been reported in children with cleft palate (McWilliams, 1969). Further, children with congenital hearing loss or hearing loss acquired in the first 2 years of life generally have voice abnormalities in conjunction with phonological and language difficulties (Wirz, 1992). Reports such as these highlight the need for a comprehensive review of associated speech, language, and hearing problems during history-taking.

Hereditary Patterns: If the patient history suggests that other family members are similarly affected, a genetic or hereditary disorder might be suspected. Although our knowledge of genetics has increased substantially in recent years, the influence of genetic factors remains obscure in many areas, including voice disorders. It is believed that the interaction between genes and the intrauterine environment can result in some congenital disorders such as cleft lip and palate (Sparks, 1984). The relationship between these factors remains controversial with respect to other speech and language areas (e.g., stuttering, motor-speech problems, and congenital laryngeal anomalies). Yet a positive family history implicates a possible genetic or hereditary component that might require special testing to ensure accurate diagnosis. In a complicated case, the interdisciplinary voice team should include a genetics counselor who can assist family members in their understanding of the underlying problem.

Case Example: Developmental and Family History/Motor-Speech Problems

Case history: This 6-year-old male was referred for voice evaluation because of concerns regarding a high-pitched speaking voice and hypernasality. According to his parents, his speech had always been difficult to understand. Delayed speech and language development was first identified through a preschool screening at age 1 and he began receiving language stimulation therapy. He had a past history of chronic serous otitis media, to which his speech and language delays had always been attributed. His family history included two older brothers with similar developmental histories and communication problems.

Observational assessment: In addition to voice, articulation, and language problems, he demonstrated coexisting problems with fluency.

Clinical hypothesis: It was hypothesized that a motor-speech disorder might underlie his multiple communication problems.

Voice evaluation: Voice evaluation, in this case, involved speech motor testing in addition to the physical examination and instrumental voice analysis. The results revealed no structural abnormalities and normal pitch and resonance during structured tasks. Poor control of the speech mechanism was demonstrated on tests of oral motor functioning; intermittent hypernasality and pitch breaks were evident during rapid, conversational speech. Overall the findings suggested that timing difficulties, secondary to motor-speech problems, were causing the disturbances in prosody and fluency as well as episodes of assimilative nasality and uncontrollable breaks in pitch.

Acceptance of the clinical hypothesis: The clinical hypothesis was accepted.

Treatment planning: It was recommended that the child continue in speech and language therapy, with a shifted emphasis toward the use of motor-speech excercises to facilitate voice control and fluency. A neurological evaluation was also recommended and the parents were counseled regarding the benefits of consultation with a genetics specialist, given the similarity of the problems in the three brothers.

The Adult History

The medical history of adults can sometimes be extremely lengthy and complex. It is not uncommon to see an elderly person, or an individual with complicated medical problems, arrive in the clinic with three or more volumes of medical charts, documenting 20, 40, 60, or even 80 years of health problems. In these cases, the clinician's first challenge is to consolidate all relevant medical, psychological, behavioral, and familial background information. The adult history questionnaire can serve as a vehicle for transporting the most pertinent information into the hands of the examiner.

The configuration of the standard adult voice history generally follows a format similar to the one shown in Table 2–3. Although each section of the history is important, four areas warrant specific discussion as their potential contributions to the voice problem might not always be easily recognized: the general medical history, effects of medications, family/work systems, and the psychological aspects of voice.

TABLE 2–3. Elements of typical adult voice history.

Voice history

Symptoms	▶ What is the chief complaint?
	▶ What changes in voice have been noticed (e.g., hoarseness, breathiness, vocal fatigue, loss of vocal range)?
	▶ Are there associated sensations (e.g., pain in the throat when vocalizing) or associated symptoms (e.g., breathing problems, swallowing difficulties, heartburn)?
Onset	▶ When did the voice problem first begin?
	▶ Was the onset sudden or gradual in nature?
	▶ What did the patient think was causing the problem?
Duration	▶ Is the problem acute (days or weeks) or chronic (months or years)?
Variability	▶ Is the problem constant or does it wax and wane?
	▶ If the problem varies, what factors seem to aggravate or relieve the symptoms (e.g., weather, amount of speaking, coughing episodes, time of day)?
Progression of symptoms	▶ Since the time of onset, have the symptoms worsened, improved, or remained the same?
	▶ What prompted evaluation?
Previous evaluations, treatments, results	▶ Have there been previous evaluations or treatments (e.g., surgery voice therapy, radiation therapy, acupuncture, homeopathy)?
	▶ What were the effects of those treatments?

Medical history

Major illnesses	▶ Have there been previous physical or mental illnesses?
	▶ What was the length of each illness, extent of incapacity, types and effects of treatments?
Surgeries	▶ What surgeries have been performed?
	▶ Was intubation or tracheostomy required?
	▶ Were there any surgical complications (e.g., recurrent laryngeal nerve section, airway obstruction, hemangioma)?
Accidents or injuries	▶ Have there been traumatic injuries to the head or neck?
	▶ Blunt or penetrating traumas (e.g., sport injuries, strangulation, automobile accidents)?
	▶ Foreign body aspiration (e.g., choking on foods or small objects)?
	▶ Ingestion of caustic agents (e.g., acids, alkalines)?
	▶ Inhalation injuries or burns?
	▶ Iatrogenic injuries (from irradiation, prolonged intubation, or tracheostomy)?
Allergies	▶ Are there allergies to foods? drugs? environment?
Review of systems	▶ Are medical symptoms present that might be associated with the voice disorder?
	▶ Are there medical conditions that might affect the specific systems (e.g., respiratory system, nervous system, intestinal system, immune system, cardiovascular system)?
	▶ Is there an identifiable symptom complex or pattern?

(continued)

TABLE 2–3. *(continued)*

Current health practices

Medications	▶ Are any drugs being used on a regular or intermittent basis? prescription drugs? nonprescription drugs (e.g., aspirin, laxatives, vitamins, cold tablets, over-the-counter sleeping pills, or nerve pills)?
Recreational drugs	▶ Is there past or present use of street drugs such as pot (marijuana), speed (amphetamines), Dexedrine, Ritalin, LSD (acid), PCP (angel dust), cocaine, heroin, mushrooms?
Tobacco	▶ What type and amount of tobacco is used?
	▶ How long has the patient been smoking or chewing tobacco?
	▶ Is the patient exposed to secondhand smoke?
Alcohol	▶ How much and what types of alcoholic beverages does the patient drink?
	▶ Are there changes in the voice symptoms with alcohol or drug consumption?
Caffeine	▶ Is there use of caffeine-containing drinks (e.g., coffee, tea, soft drinks, hot chocolate)? foods (e.g., chocolate bars, cocoa), or medications (e.g., Excedrin™, Anacin™, Vanquish™, Triaminicin™, Coricidin™, Sinarest™, No-Doz™, diet pills)?
Dietary patterns	▶ Is there a special or restricted diet?
	▶ Would the present diet promote gastroesophageal reflux (e.g., spicy foods, high-fat foods, caffeine)?
	▶ Is there evidence of an eating disorder such as anorexia nervosa or bulimia?
Voice usage	▶ In what ways is the voice typically used (e.g., cheering at a sports events, professional or public speaking, talking over noise in a factory, singing, yodeling, crying)?
Stress management	▶ In what ways is stress managed (e.g., exercise, medication, counseling, meditation, support groups, primal scream therapy)?

Family/work history

Hereditary conditions	▶ What inheritance patterns are present in the family history?
	▶ Are there similar problems in parents, siblings, offspring?
Family dynamics/Learning	▶ Do environmental influences seem to account for the voice problem (e.g., is the patient from a large family that "always talked too loudly")?
	▶ What current family interaction patterns exist (e.g., shouting matches, verbal competition at the dinner table)?
Major life changes	▶ What events have happened in the past 12 months that might increase stress?
Emotional reactions to illness	▶ Is the patient's reaction to illness normal or extreme (e.g., too blase; too frightened)?
	▶ Is there a family history of "throat cancer"?
	▶ Is overreaction to the current voice problem based on past family experiences?

(continued)

TABLE 2–3. *(continued)*

Psychological considerations	
Psychological history	▸ What is the patient's mental health history?
	▸ Does it include depression, mania, suicide attempts, alcohol abuse, an eating disorder, schizophrenia, "nervous breakdowns," sexual abuse, or other psychological problems?
	▸ What past or present treatments have been used (e.g., psychotherapy, pharmacotherapy, electroconvulsive therapy, inpatient hospitalizations)?
Current stress levels	▸ Have recent problems or circumstances elevated stress levels at home or work (e.g., financial problems, divorce, illness or death in the family, change in jobs, moving to a new city)?
Voice disability index	▸ What impact is the voice problem having on daily living activities?

The General Medical History: Because the body is composed of different groups of organs that work together to perform one or more vital functions (e.g., the respiratory system, the musculoskeletal system, the cardiovascular system, the gastrointestinal system), health problems in one system can often affect another system; it is common for illnesses in various systems to impact on the voice. This is particularly true of multisystemic conditions (e.g., systemic lupus erythematosus) where the body may be generally affected by a disease process. Although this concept is familiar to health care professionals, patients might not understand the possible relationship between their gastrointestinal problems and hoarseness, or their emphysema and loudness. As a consequence, many general health or medical problems can go unreported unless a review of systems survey (similar to the one in Table 2–4) is incorporated into the history questionnaire.

A review of systems survey (Table 2–4) is a symptomatology checklist that can aid voice clinicians in relating systemic diseases and general health problems to changes in the voice. For example, the presence of joint pain and swelling in the hands, wrists, and knees, along with vocal fold stiffness and/ or reduced arytenoid movement, would alert the clinician to the possibility of an inflammatory disease such as systemic lupus erythematosus (SLE) or rhematoid arthritis of the larynx. A second cluster of symptoms, namely, facial pain, headache, nonspecific throat discomfort, foreign body sensation, odynophagia, and increased salivation might suggest Eagle's syndrome, a head and neck syndrome that can affect voice when there is irritation to branches of the cranial nerves (V, VII, IX, X) due to elongation and ossification of the styloid process.

Many systemic and multisystemic conditions can affect voice, including acromegaly, hypothyroidism, thyroid nodules, parathyroid dysfunction, ovarian cysts, Cushing's syndrome, gastroesophageal reflux, monilia, asthma, arthritis, mumps, lupus, gout, Sjogren's syndrome, Arnold Chiari malformation, amyloidosis, scleroma, Werner's syndrome, herpes, gonorrhea, syphilis, diabetes mellitus, renal insufficiency, degenerative neurological diseases, tuberculosis, Wegener's granulomatosis, and porphyria. The medical symptoms of selected illnesses are summarized in Chapter 3.

The variety of laryngeal manifestations seen in patients with systemic or multisystemic diseases is also great. Associated voice and laryngeal findings might include mucosal ulceration, nodularity, diffuse in-

TABLE 2–4. Review of systems.

HAVE YOU BEEN TROUBLED OR ARE YOU TROUBLED NOW BY ANY OF THE FOLLOWING?

GENERAL:	Yes	No	SKELETON AND JOINTS:	Yes	No
Excessive fatigue	____	____	Swollen or painful joints	____	____
Unexplained weight change	____	____	Neck pains	____	____
Excessive thirst	____	____	Gout	____	____
Intolerance for hot weather	____	____	Frequent back stiffness	____	____
Unexplainable perspiration	____	____	Back trouble	____	____
Persistent pain in any part of the body	____	____	Severe leg cramps	____	____
Lumps or swelling	____	____	Difficulty walking	____	____
Exercise related health or breathing problems	____	____	INTESTINAL SYSTEM:		
			Change in eating habits	____	____
SKIN AND HAIR:			Frequent indigestion	____	____
Recurrent skin rash	____	____	Heartburn	____	____
Recurrent sores	____	____	Frequent belching	____	____
Patches of hair falling out	____	____	Recurrent abdominal pain	____	____
Swollen glands	____	____	Frequent nausea or vomiting	____	____
Excessive coarseness of hair	____	____	Bitter or acid taste in mouth	____	____
Persistent or recurrent itching	____	____	NERVOUS SYSTEM:		
Excessive dryness of skin	____	____	Frequent or severe headaches	____	____
EYE, EAR, NOSE & THROAT:			Attacks of staggering or loss of balance	____	____
Facial pain	____	____	Unexplained dizziness	____	____
Blurred or double vision	____	____	Loss of consciousness	____	____
Loss of vision	____	____	Head injury	____	____
Loss of hearing	____	____	Weakness or heaviness of limbs	____	____
Ringing in ears	____	____	Persistent or recurrent numbness or tingling of hands or feet	____	____
Ear pain	____	____	Episodes of difficulty talking	____	____
Trouble with nose or sinuses	____	____	Increasing irritability and mood swings	____	____
Teeth or gum problems	____	____	Prolonged periods of feeling depressed or blue	____	____
Voice changes	____	____	Difficulty in concentrating	____	____
Swallowing problems	____	____	Difficulty in memorizing	____	____
HEART:			Difficulty in sleeping	____	____
Abnormal chest x-ray	____	____	Uncontrollable tension	____	____
Chest pain	____	____	Twitching or tremors	____	____
Discomfort in chest on exertion	____	____	Personal problems that cause you great concern	____	____
Palpitation of the heart	____	____	Suicidal thoughts	____	____
Heart murmur	____	____	GENITOURINARY:		
Other heart trouble	____	____	Gonorrhea or syphilis	____	____
Leg cramps while walking	____	____	Herpes	____	____
Ankle swelling	____	____	(Women only)		
High blood pressure	____	____	Possibly pregnant	____	____
RESPIRATORY:			Change in menstrual pattern	____	____
Sleep apnea	____	____	Other menstrual problems	____	____
Cough	____	____	IMMUNE SYSTEM:		
Sputum (phlegm) production	____	____	Unexplained bruising	____	____
Pneumonia or pleurisy	____	____	Lymph nodes swelling or pain	____	____
Shortness of breath with activity	____	____	HIV positive	____	____
Wheezing or asthma	____	____	Other immunologic problems	____	____
Pulmonary emboli (blood clot to the lung)	____	____			
Exposure to toxic dusts, chemicals	____	____			

Source: Adapted by Koschkee (1994) from the Allergy Clinic Intake Form, UW Hospital and Clinics, Madison, Wisconsin.

flammation, laryngeal edema, vocal fold hyperplasia, fixation or dysfunction of the cricoarytenoid joint, vocal fold paralysis, epiglottitis, or other laryngeal alterations. Uncovering the pathophysiology of voice problems such as these requires a careful review of both the signs (physical evidence of disease) and symptoms (subjective evidence of disease).

Family/Work Systems: Contemporary assessment methodology emphasizes the importance of viewing the patient not as an isolated entity, but rather as an integral part of his or her family system and work system. When the assessment of voice disorders is approached from this perspective, factors or circumstances that might affect all family members (e.g., caring for a spouse with a debilitating physical illness or chronic depression, living in a household with chronic

vocal abuse, or having a close relative who has recently died of cancer) or that might impinge on the patient in the work environment (e.g., conflict with a coworker, change in job responsibilities) are considered significant parts of the voice history.

In considering the patient's family systems, it is important to recognize that the illnesses of other family members might influence patients' reactions to their own voice problems. For instance, it is common to see patients seeking evaluation in the clinic because of concerns about throat cancer. Often these individuals have a family history of cancer, perhaps even laryngeal cancer. In these situations, an exaggerated concern about the voice problem may develop. Knowing about the medical history of close relatives (Table 2–5) can assist, not only in identifying hereditary conditions, but also in understanding the patient's re-

TABLE 2–5. Family history.

	Yes	No	Unsure	Who (e.g., mother, brother, aunt, etc.)
Please indicate if any family members have had any of the following illnesses. If so, who?				
Heart disease				
High blood pressure				
Stroke				
Cancer				
Alcoholism				
Drug abuse				
Thyroid disorder				
Seizures (epilepsy)				
Migraines				
Allergies				
Asthma				
Ulcers				
Depression				
Neurologic disease				
Psychiatric problems				
Other (please list)				

action to illness. Other potential sources of stress, related to either changes within the family or work setting, can usually be established by including a life change survey (Table 2–6). This type of survey asks patients to identify major life events that have happened to them in the last 12 months.

Psychological Aspects of Voice: Establishing the relationship between the mind and body frequently becomes the center of the adult's history because similiar symptoms may occur due to physical illness or psychological distress. For example, a monotonous voice can signify fatigue or depression. Rapid rate can relate to a neurological problem or to anxiety. Feeling a "lump in the throat" could result from gastroesophageal reflux or from fear. Hoarseness may be caused by a mass lesion on the vocal folds or dry mucosa, an anxiety response of the sympathetic nervous system. Consequently, probes into an individual's personality, present psychological state, and psychological history are crucial elements of the voice history. If information is needed that extends beyond the standard voice history, supplemental questionnaires such as the Millon Behavioral Inventory (Table 2–7) or the Beck Depression Inventory (Table 2–8) can be used as screening devices to assist in differential diagnosis and/or aid in the identification of problems in need of psychological referral.

Another useful measure, the Voice Disability Index (Appendix 2–1) (Koschkee, 1993), assists in determining the degree of disability perceived by the individual in home, work, and social situations. This psychodynamic measure attempts to reflect,

TABLE 2–6. Life change survey.

Family/Work Systems:

What events have happened to you in the past 12 months? Please check those that apply.

Death of spouse	☐
Divorce	☐
Marital difficulties/separation	☐
Change in health of family member	☐
Death of family member	☐
Death of close friend	☐
Fired from job	☐
Personal injury or illness	☐
Change in financial state	☐
Change in living conditions	☐
Change in responsibilities at work	☐
Trouble with boss or coworker	☐
Sexual difficulties	☐
Retirement	☐
Other	☐
(specify other: _____)	

TABLE 2–7. Examples from the Million Behavioral Health Inventory.

T	F	I often feel so angry that I want to throw and break things.
T	F	I get so touchy that I can't talk about certain things.
T	F	I always take the medicine a doctor tells me to even if I don't think it is working.

Source: From the *Million Behavioral Health Inventory.* Copyright 1976; 1981 by Dr. Theodore Million. Portions reproduced by permission of the publisher, National Computer Systems, Inc., Minnetonka, Minnesota. All rights reserved.

TABLE 2–8. Examples from the Beck Depression Inventory.

0	I do not feel sad.
1	I feel sad.
2	I am sad all the time and I can't snap out of it.
3	I am so sad or unhappy that I can't stand it.
0	I don't cry anymore than usual.
1	I cry more now than I used to.
2	I cry all the time now.
3	I used to cry, but now I can't cry, even though I want to.

Source: From the *Beck Depression Inventory.* Copyright 1978 by Aaron T. Beck. Reproduced by permission of the publisher, The Psychological Corporation, San Antonio, Texas. All rights reserved.

from the patient's perspective, the impact that the voice problem has on daily life. It also serves to document perceived vocal disability pre- and post-treatment. It is particularly useful in cases where vocal effort or fatigue predominate, as in milder cases of spasmodic dysphonia or presbylaryngis.

Medications: The patient's use of medications requires special consideration, because the side effects of drugs may produce adverse reactions on the voice. Colton and Casper (1990), Fried (1988), and Martin (1992) have discussed some of the direct effects of drugs on phonation, such as drying of the laryngeal mucosa, disruption of coordination and proprioception, structural changes (e.g., vocal fold bowing), and involuntary laryngeal movements. There are also some indirect or secondary effects of drug use that can contribute to voice problems. For instance, some medications, including certain drugs used to reduce hypertension, trigger abusive habits or laryngeal behaviors, such as chronic coughing, that can irritate the larynx. Manuals such as the *Physician's Desk Reference* (PDR) (1996), and the *Compendium of Pharmaceuticals and Specialties* (CPS) assist clinicians in identifying both the direct and the indirect effects of medications.

Voice specialists also need to recognize that members of the geriatric population are at greater risk for developing voice changes related to medication use. Because the incidence of health problems increases with age, elderly individuals are more likely to take medications than their younger counterparts. Braunwald et al. (1987) estimate that approximately 90% of the geriatric population take at least one type of medication, and the majority take two or more medications concurrently, a practice referred to as "polypharmacy." When patients use different medications to treat multiple problems, the chances for adverse drug-to-drug interactions increase substantially, particularly in older persons who metabolize drugs less predictably.

Case Example: Medication
Effects/Chronic Hypertrophic Laryngitis

Case History: This 65-year-old retired high school history teacher came into the Voice Clinic complaining of intermittent hoarseness, and "froggy voice," especially in the mornings. He had been referred to Otolaryngology by a physician in the General Medicine Clinic who was seeing the patient for treatment of a chronic cough. The patient stated that he had contracted a "head cold" 6 months earlier that had left him with a persistent, dry, hacking cough and hoarseness. He was treated with an antibiotic for 1 month, without change. Allergy testing, chest x-rays, and pulmonary function testing had proven negative. The patient's only medication was a high blood pressure medicine that he reported taking for over 25 years. Occasional symptoms of gastroesophageal reflux were described.

Observational assessment: The patient was observed to cough frequently during the evaluation. No other observations were considered significant.

Clinical hypothesis: It was hypothesized that the patient's chronic coughing was producing the dysphonia; it was also hypothesized that his chronic cough was due to gastroesophageal reflux as the other most common causes for coughing—postnasal drip, asthma, and chronic bronchitis—had already been ruled out, and the patient was experiencing some reflux symptoms.

Instrumental evaluation: During laryngeal examination and videostroboscopy, both vocal folds were observed to have a slightly polypoid and thickened appearance. There were no lesions seen in the hypopharynx or larynx and normal mobility was present bilaterally. His physiological f_0 range was slightly compromised, acoustic perturbation levels in speech were high due to a tendency to use glottal fry register, and maximum phonation time fell below the expected value of 15 seconds. The impression was chronic hypertrophic laryngitis secondary to the chronic cough.

Indecision about the hypothesis: Although the instrumental measures of voice were consistent with an etiology of chronic coughing, additional testing was needed to determine that the coughing was secondary to gastroesophageal reflux.

Collateral testing: Following a consultation with the internist, the patient was referred to the gastroenterology clinic for reflux evaluation. Esophageal pH monitoring was conducted, but the findings were negative. These results prompted the voice care team to reevaluate their clinical hypothesis.

Regeneration of an alternate hypothesis: Although the relationship between the coughing episodes and the patient's dysphonia appeared obvious to both the patient and the examiners, the etiology of the cough was not. The culprit—Prinivil® (lisinopril), a hypertension medication that sometimes produces cough as a side-effect —was discovered following a more careful review of the written history. Although the clinicians had initially suspected a relationship between the hypertension medication and the persistent coughing, the patient had reported taking his high-blood-pressure medicine for over 25 years. He had neglected to mention, and the examiners had neglected to ask, if a change in medication had occurred within the past year. Only the history form had asked, "How long have you been taking this particular drug?" Indeed, the patient had recently been switched to a new drug. When the dates between the onset of his problems and the medication change corresponded, the etiology was recognized. The coughing episodes were eliminated and the voice improved when his internist prescribed a different drug to treat the hypertension.

The Personal Interview

Questionnaires, however informative, can never replace the direct, face-to-face interaction that occurs in the personal interview. From the patient's perspective, the personal interview is a time to elaborate more fully on important aspects of the case history, to express feelings and concerns about the voice problem, and to respond to any troublesome questions on the written questionnaire. For the examiner, the personal interview offers an opportunity to learn about the patient in greater depth, make auditory-perceptual judgments of the patient's voice, and begin the observational assessment process.

As a general rule, open-ended questions both begin and end a history interview. The clinician might open the session with:

What brings you to our clinic today? or How can I help you?

Given the opportunity, many patients communicate their most vital concerns within the first few statements:

My voice has been hoarse for over 2 months and I stopped smoking but it's no better. Do you think I have cancer? My dad died of cancer, you know. or, I've had problems with my voice since they put a tube down my throat two years ago after my heart attack. My family doctor says they probably damaged my voice box.

Throughout the body of the interview, questions become more specific in nature as the clinician relates reported behaviors or symptoms to possible etiologies and begins to develop a clinical hypothesis about the pathogenesis of the voice disorder. As an example, in a case where an older patient is exhibiting signs of essential voice tremor, the clinician might probe into the family history for evidence of other neurological problems because heredity can play a role in the development of a voice tremor:

You mentioned that your aunt has a voice that is similar to yours. How are your voices similar? . . . So you've noticed shakiness in her voice, too. Have you ever noticed "shakiness" in any other part of her body? . . . You have been aware of a head tremor? Do you know if your aunt has been seen by a neurologist? What did the neurologist tell your aunt about her voice problem?

At the conclusion of the interview, it is advisable to return to a final open-ended question:

Is there anything we haven't discussed that you feel is important?

Surprisingly, the percentage of positive responses is quite high, and sometimes important information is conveyed. Some patients feel more comfortable disclosing personal information at the end of the interview after trust and rapport have been established. In one case, a quiet adult patient who stuttered and also had voice problems was being seen because of a feeling of "constriction" and "tightness" in the laryngeal area. When asked at the end of the interview if he had anything else to add, he responded,

Well, maybe. Did I mention that I was hung from a tree as a child?

In a second instance, a 33-year-old accountant revealed at the end of a case history interview that his "real" reason for seeking evaluation was not a fear of public speaking, as he had led the examiners to believe, but rather his concerns about his transexualism.

Of course, interviewing style and technique are critical determinants of the interview outcome. Since most speech pathology and medical interns feel insecure initially about the diagnostic interview, instructors constantly search for resources to offer their students-in-training. Billings and Stoeckle (1989) provide a step-by-step guide to successful medical interviewing. This book is an excellent resource for student interns and portions are a worthwhile review for seasoned practitioners. Coulehan and Block (1992), Lumsden and Whiteside (1987), and

Enelow and Swisher (1986) also offer assistive primers that detail the medical interview process. Sataloff (1991) provides an excellent review of the professional voice users' history. Other authors—Aronson (1990), Boone and McFarlane (1994), Colton and Casper (1990), Ford and Bless (1991), Greene and Mathieson (1989), Prater and Swift (1989), Stemple (1984), and Wilson (1979)—review the voice history from a speech pathology perspective. Of these, Wilson (1979) discusses the pediatric history. Morrison and Rammage et al. (1994) provide an interdisciplinary perspective on personal interviewing that includes approaches to obtaining psychological aspects of the history. More detailed instruction on the psychiatric interview can be found in Shea (1988).

The practiced interviewer will also be more adept in the corollary exercise of informal observational assessment, for observational assessment (like diagnostic interviewing) integrates both the scientific and the artistic aspects of voice care. A discussion of the art of observational assessment follows.

REFERENCES

Aronson, A. E. (1990). *Clinical voice disorders: An interdisciplinary approach* (3rd ed.). New York: Thieme-Stratton Inc.

Batch, A. J. (1988). *ENT manifestation of reflux.* American Academy of Otolaryngology—Head and Neck Surgery, Inc.

Baumgartner, J. M., Ramig, L. A., & Kuehn, D. P. (1986). Voice disorders and stuttering in children. In T. J. Balkany & N. R. T. Dashley (Eds.), *Clinical pediatric otolaryngology.* St. Louis, MO: C. V. Mosby.

Beck, A. T. (1978). *Beck depression inventory.* San Antonio, TX: Psychological Corp.

Billings, J. A., & Stoeckle, J. D. (1989). *The clinical encounter: A guide to the medical interview and case presentation.* Chicago: Year Book Medical Publishers, Inc.

Bless, D. M. (1994). *Vocal cord dysfunction patient history form.* Madison: University of Wisconsin Hospital and Clinics.

Bless, D. M., & Ford, C. N. (1989). *Spasmodic dysphonia study: Demographic data and history questionnaire.* Madison: University of Wisconsin Hospital and Clinics.

Boone, D. R., & McFarlane, S. C. (1994). *The voice and voice therapy* (5th ed.). Englewood Cliffs, NJ: Prentice-Hall.

Braunwald, E., Isselbacher, K. J., Petersdorf, R. G., Wilson, J. D., Martin, J. B., & Fauci, A. S. (1987). *Harrison's principles of internal medicine* (11th ed.). New York: McGraw-Hill Book Company.

Burton, D. M., Pransky, S. M., Kearns, D.B., Katz, R. M., & Seid, A .B. (1992). Pediatric airway manifestations of gastroesophageal reflux. *Annals of Otology, Rhinology and Laryngology, 101*(9), 742–749.

Carlson, K. A. (1992, July). *Recognition of voice disorders in children.* Paper presented at the Phonosurgery Symposium, Madison, WI.

Castle, D. L. (1982). *Signaling and assistive listening devices for hearing-impaired people.* Alexander Graham Bell Association for the Deaf.

Colton, R. H., & Casper, J. K. (1990). *Understanding voice problems: A physiological perspective for diagnosis and treatment.* Baltimore: Wilkins & Wilkins.

Compendium of Pharmaceuticals and Specialties (32nd ed.). (1997). Ottawa: Canadian Pharmaceutical Association.

Contencin, P., & Narcy, P. (1992). Gastropharyngeal reflux in infants and children: A pharyngeal pH monitoring study. *Archives of Otolaryngology—Head Neck Surgery, 118,* 1028–1030.

Coulehan, J. L., & Block, M. R. (1992). The medical interview: A primer for students of the art (2nd ed.). Philadelphia: F. A. Davis.

Earnest, D. L. (1991, September). *Atypical manifestations of gastroesophageal reflux.* Paper presented at the American Academy of Otolaryngology Conference.

Enelow, A. J., & Swisher, S. N. (1986). *Interviewing and patient care* (3rd ed.). New York: Oxford University Press.

Ford, C. N., & Bless, D. M. (1991). Phonosurgery: Assessment and surgical management of voice disorders. New York: Raven Press.

Fried, M. P. (1988). *The larynx: A multidisciplinary approach.* Boston: Little, Brown.

Gray, S. D. (1992, July). *Treatment of pediatric laryngeal disorders.* Paper presented at the Phonosurgery Symposium, Madison, WI.

Greene, M. C. L., & Mathieson, L. (1989). The voice and its disorders (5th ed.). San Diego: Singular Publishing Group.

Heatley, D. (1992). In-service presented to Department of Surgery, University of Wisconsin Hospital and Clinics, University of Wisconsin-Madison, Madison.

Jones, N. S., Lannigan, F. J., McCullagh, M., Anggiansah, A., Owen, W., & Harris, T. M. (1990). Acid reflux and hoarseness. *Journal of Voice, 4*, 355–358.

Koschkee, D. C. (1993). *Voice disability index.* Madison, WI: University of Wisconsin Hospital and Clinics.

Laver, J., & Mackenzie-Beck, J. (1992). *Vocal profile analysis course.* Madison, WI.

Lumsden, C. J., & Whiteside, C. I. (1987). Clinical methods. New York: Alan R. Liss.

Martin, F. G. (1992, November). *Drugs and voice.* Paper presented at the American Speech and Hearing Convention, San Antonio, TX.

McWilliams, B. J. (1969). Diagnostic implications of vocal fold nodules in children with cleft palate. *Laryngoscope, 79*, 2072–2080.

Million, T. (1976/1981). *Million Behavioral Inventory,* Minnetonka, MN: National Computer Systems, Inc.

Morrison, M., & Rammage, L., with Nichol, H., Pullan, B., May, P., & Salkeld, L. (1994) *The management of voice disorders.* London: Chapman & Hall Medical.

Olson, N. R. (1991). Laryngopharyngeal manifestations of gastroesophageal reflux disease. *Otolaryngologic Clinics of North America, 24*(5).

Physician's desk reference (50th ed.). (1996). Oradell, NJ: Medical Economics Co.

Prater, R. J., & Swift, R. W. (1989). *Manual of voice therapy* (2nd ed.). Boston.

Sataloff, R. T. (1991). *Professional voice: The science and art of clinical care.* New York: Raven Press.

Sataloff, R. T. (1997). *Professional voice: The science and art of clinical care* (2nd ed.). San Diego: Singular Publishing Group.

Shea, S. C. (1988). *Psychiatric interviewing: The art of understanding.* Philadelphia: W. B. Saunders.

Shriberg, L. D., Kwiatkowski, J., Best, S., Hengst, J., & Terselic-Weber, B. (1986). Characteristics of children with phonologic disorders of unknown origin. *Journal of Speech and Hearing Disorders, 51*(2).

Sparks, S. N. (1984). *Birth defects and speech-language disorders.* San Diego: College-Hill Press.

Stemple, J. C. (1984). *Clinical voice pathology: Theory and management.* Columbus, OH: Charles E. Merrill.

St. Louis, K. O., Hansen, G., Buch, J., & Oliver, J. L. (1992). Voice deviations and coexisting communication disorders. *Language, Speech and Hearing Services in the Schools, 23*(1), 82–87.

St. Louis, K. O., & Hinzman, A. R. (1988). A descriptive study of speech, language, and hearing characteristics of school-aged stutterers. *Journal of Fluency Disorders, 40*, 211–215.

Wilson, D. K. (1979). *Voice problems of children* (3rd ed.). Baltimore: Williams & Wilkins.

Wilson, J. A., White, A., Haacke, N. P., Maran, A. G. D., Heading, R. C., Pryde, A., & Piris, J. (1989). Gastroesophageal reflux and posterior laryngitis. *Annals of Otology, Rhinology and Laryngology, 98*(6), 405–410.

Wirz, S. (1992). The voice of the deaf. In M. Fawcus (Ed.), *Voice disorders and their management* (2nd ed.). San Diego: Singular Publishing Group.

APPENDIX 2–1

Voice Disability Index

Name _____ Date _____

INSTRUCTIONS: First, mark on the line where appropriate. Then circle the closest corresponding number.

Work

Because of my voice problems, my work is impaired

1	2	3	4	5	6	7

Not at all   Mildly   Moderately   Markedly   Very Severely

Social Life/Leisure Activities

Because of my voice problems, my social life/leisure time is impaired

1	2	3	4	5	6	7

Not at all   Mildly   Moderately   Markedly   Very Severely

Family Life/Home Responsibilities

Because of my voice problems, my family life/home responsibilities are impaired

1	2	3	4	5	6	7

Not at all   Mildly   Moderately   Markedly   Very Severely

Adapted by Koschkee (1993) from Disability Scale, Psychiatry Clinic, University of Wisconsin Hospital and Clinics, Madison, Wisconsin.

APPENDIX 2–2

Patient History: Singers[1]

Robert Thayer Sataloff, M.D., D.M.A.
1721 Pine Street
Philadelphia, PA 19103
U.S.A.

NAME _____ AGE _____ SEX _____ RACE _____

HEIGHT _____ WEIGHT _____ DATE _____

VOICE CATEGORY: _____ soprano   _____ mezzo-soprano   _____ alto

                     _____ tenor   _____ baritone   _____ bass

(If you are not currently having a voice problem, please skip to Question #3.)

PLEASE CHECK OR CIRCLE CORRECT ANSWERS

1. How long have you had your present voice problem?

    Who noticed it?

    [self, family, voice teacher, critics, everyone, other _____]

    Do you know what caused it?   Yes _____   No _____

    If yes, what?   .

    Did it come on slowly or suddenly?   Slowly _____   Suddenly _____
    Is it getting: Worse: _____ , Better _____ , Same _____

2. Which symptoms do you have? (Please check all that apply.)
    _____ Hoarseness (coarse or scratchy sound)
    _____ Fatigue (voice tires or changes quality after singing for a short period of time)
    _____ Volume disturbance (trouble singing)   softly _____   loudly _____
    _____ Loss of range (high _____   low _____)
    _____ Change in classification (example: voice lowered from soprano to mezzo)
    _____ Prolonged warm-up time (over ½ hr to warm up voice)
    _____ Breathiness
    _____ Tickling or choking sensation while singing
    _____ Pain in throat while singing
    _____ Other: (Please specify)_____
    _____
    _____
    _____

3. Do you have an important performance soon?   Yes _____   No _____
        Date(s): _____

[1]From Sataloff, R. T. (1997). Professional Voice: *The Art and Science of Clinical Care* (2nd ed., pp. 832–844). San Diego: Singular Publishing Group. Reprinted with permission.

4. What is the current status of your singing career?
    Professional _____   Amateur _____

5. What are your long-term career goals in singing?
    [   ] Premiere operatic career
    [   ] Premiere pop music career
    [   ] Active avocation
    [   ] Classical
    [   ] Pop
    [   ] Other (_____)
    [   ] Amateur performance (choral or solo)
    [   ] Amateur singing for own pleasure

6. Have you had voice training?   Yes _____   No _____
    At what age did you begin?

7. Have there been periods of months or years without lessons in that time?
    Yes _____   No _____

8. How long have you studied with your present teacher?

    Teacher's name:
    Teacher's address:

    Teacher's telephone number:

9. Please list previous teachers and years during which you studied with them.

10. Have you ever had training for your speaking voice?   Yes _____   No _____
    Acting voice lessons?   Yes _____   No _____
    How many years?
    Speech therapy?   Yes _____   No _____
    How many months?

11. Do you have a job in addition to singing?   Yes _____   No _____

    If yes, does it involve extensive voice use?   Yes _____   No _____

    If yes, what is it? [actor, announcer (television/radio/sports arena), athletic instructor, attorney, clergy, politician, physician, salesperson, stockbroker, teacher, telephone operator or receptionist, waiter, waitress, secretary, other _____

12. In your performance work, in addition to singing, are you frequently
    required to speak?   Yes _____   No _____
    dance?   Yes _____   No _____

13. How many years did you sing actively before beginning voice lessons initially?

14. What types of music do you sing? (Check all that apply.)
    _____ Classical   _____ Show
    _____ Nightclub   _____ Rock
    _____ Other: (Please specify.) _____
    _____

15. Do you regularly sing in a sitting position (such as from behind a piano or drum set)?
    Yes _____   No _____

16. Do you sing outdoors or in large halls, or with orchestras? (Circle which one.)
    Yes _____   No _____

17. If you perform with electrical instruments or outdoors, do you use monitor speakers?
    Yes _____   No _____

    If yes, can you hear them?   Yes _____   No _____

18. Do you play a musical instrument(s)?   Yes _____   No _____
    If yes, please check all that apply:
    _____ Keyboard (piano, organ, harpsichord, other _____)
    _____ Violin, viola
    _____ Cello
    _____ Bass
    _____ Plucked strings (guitar, harp, other _____)
    _____ Brass
    _____ Wind with single reed
    _____ Wind with double reed
    _____ Flute, piccolo
    _____ Percussion
    _____ Bagpipe
    _____ Accordion
    _____ Other: (Please specify.)_____

19. How often do you practice?
    Scales: [daily, few times weekly, once a week, rarely, never]

    If you practice scales, do you do them all at once, or do you divide them up over the course of a day? [all at once, two or three sittings]

    On days when you do scales, how long do you practice them?
    [15,30,45,60,75,90,105,120, more] minutes

    Songs: [daily, few times weekly, once a week, rarely, never]

    How many hours per day?
    [½,1,1½,2,2½,3,more]

Do you warm up your voice before you sing?   Yes _____   No _____

Do you warm down your voice when you finish singing?   Yes _____   No _____

20. How much are you singing at present (total including practice time) (average hours per day)?

    Rehearsal: _____

    Performance: _____

21. Please check all that apply to you:

    _____ Voice worse in the morning

    _____ Voice worse later in the day, after it has been used

    _____ Sing performances or rehearsals in the morning

    _____ Speak extensively (e.g., teacher, clergy, attorney, telephone work)

    _____ Cheerleader

    _____ Speak extensively backstage or at postperformance parties

    _____ Choral conductor

    _____ Frequently clear your throat

    _____ Frequent sore throat

    _____ Jaw joint problems

    _____ Bitter or acid taste, or bad breath first thing in the morning

    _____ Frequent "heartburn" or hiatal hernia

    _____ Frequent yelling or loud talking

    _____ Frequent whispering

    _____ Chronic fatigue (insomnia)

    _____ Work around extreme dryness

    _____ Frequent exercise (weight lifting, aerobics)

    _____ Frequently thirsty, dehydrated

    _____ Hoarseness first thing in the morning

    _____ Chest cough

    _____ Eat late at night

    _____ Ever used antacids

    _____ Under particular stress at present (personal or professional)

    _____ Frequent bad breath

    _____ Live, work, or perform around smoke or fumes

    _____ Traveled recently: When: _____

                                 Where: _____

    Eat any of the following before singing?

    _____ Chocolate   _____ Coffee

    _____ Alcohol   _____ Milk or ice cream

    _____ Nuts   _____ Spiced foods

    Other: (Please specify.)

    _____ Any specific vocal technical difficulties? [trouble singing soft, trouble singing loud, poor pitch control, support problems, problems at register transitions, other] Describe other:

_____ Any problems with your singing voice recently prior to the onset of the problem that brought you here? [hoarseness, breathiness, fatigue, loss of range, voice breaks, pain singing, other] Describe other:

_____ Any voice problems in the past that required a visit to a physician? If yes, please describe problem(s) and treatment(s): [laryngitis, nodules, polyps, hemorrhage, cancer, other] Describe other:

22. Your family doctor's name, address, and telephone number:

23. Your laryngologist's name, address, and telephone number:

24. Recent cold?   Yes _____   No _____

25. Current cold?   Yes _____   No _____

26. Have you been exposed to any of the following chemicals frequently (or recently) at home or at work? (Check all that apply.)

_____ Carbon monoxide   _____ Arsenic
_____ Mercury   _____ Aniline dyes
_____ Insecticides   _____ Industrial solvents (benzene, etc.)
_____ Lead   _____ Stage smoke

27. Have you been evaluated by an allergist?   Yes _____   No _____

If yes, what allergies do you have:
[none, dust, mold, trees, cats, dogs, foods, other]
(Medication allergies are covered elsewhere in this history form.)
If yes, give name and address of allergist:

28. How many packs of cigarettes do you smoke per day?

Smoking history
_____ Never
_____ Quit. When? _____
_____ Smoked about _____ packs per day for _____ years.
_____ Smoke _____ packs per day. Have smoked for _____ years.

29. Do you work or live in a smoky environment?   Yes _____   No _____

30. How much alcohol do you drink? [none, rarely, a few times per week, daily]
    If daily, or few times per week, on the average, how much do you consume?
    [1,2,3,4,5,6,7,8,9,10, more] glasses per [day, week] of [beer, wine, liquor].

    Did you formerly drink more heavily?   Yes _____   No _____

31. How many cups of coffee, tea, cola, or other caffeine-containing drinks do you drink per day?

32. List other recreational drugs you use [marijuana, cocaine, amphetamines, barbiturates, heroin, other]:

33. Have you noticed any of the following? (Check all that apply)
    _____ Hypersensitivity to heat or cold
    _____ Excessive sweating
    _____ Change in weight: gained/lost _____ lb in _____
                            weeks/ _____ months
    _____ Change in skin or hair
    _____ Palpitation (fluttering) of the heart
    _____ Emotional lability (swings of mood)
    _____ Double vision
    _____ Numbness of the face or extremities
    _____ Tingling around the mouth or face
    _____ Blurred vision or blindness
    _____ Weakness or paralysis of the face
    _____ Clumsiness in arms or legs
    _____ Confusion or loss of consciousness
    _____ Difficulty with speech
    _____ Difficulty with swallowing
    _____ Seizure (epileptic fit)
    _____ Pain in the neck or shoulder
    _____ Shaking or tremors
    _____ Memory change
    _____ Personality change

    For females:

Are you pregnant?	Yes _____	No _____
Are your menstrual periods regular?	Yes _____	No _____
Have you undergone hysterectomy?	Yes _____	No _____
Were your ovaries removed?	Yes _____	No _____
At what age did you reach puberty?	Yes _____	No _____
Have you gone through menopause?	Yes _____	No _____

    If yes, when?

34. Have you ever consulted a psychologist or psychiatrist?   Yes _____   No _____

    Are you currently under treatment?   Yes _____   No _____

35. Have you injured your head or neck (whiplash, etc.)?   Yes _____   No _____

36. Describe any serious accidents related to this visit.
    None _____

37. Are you involved in legal action involving problems with your voice?
    Yes _____   No _____

38. List names of spouse and children:

39. Brief summary of ear, nose, and throat (ENT) problems, some of which may not be related to your present complaint.

    PLEASE CHECK ALL THAT APPLY

    _____ Hearing loss   _____ Ear pain
    _____ Ear noises   _____ Facial pain
    _____ Dizziness   _____ Stiff neck
    _____ Facial paralysis   _____ Lump in neck
    _____ Nasal obstruction   _____ Lump in face or head
    _____ Nasal deformity   _____ Trouble swallowing
    _____ Mouth sores   _____ Excess eye skin
    _____ Jaw joint problem   _____ Excess facial skin
    _____ Eye problem
    _____ Other: (Please specify.)

40. Do you have or have you ever had:
    _____ Diabetes   _____ Other illnesses: (Please specify.)
    _____ Hypoglycemia   _____ Seizures
    _____ Thyroid problems   _____ Psychiatric therapy
    _____ Syphilis   _____ Frequent bad headaches
    _____ Gonorrhea   _____ Ulcers
    _____ Herpes   _____ Kidney disease
    _____ Cold sores (fever blisters)   _____ Urinary problems
    _____ High blood pressure   _____ Arthritis or skeletal problems
    _____ Severe low blood pressure   _____ Cleft palate
    _____ Intravenous antibiotics or diuretics   _____ Asthma
    _____ Heart attack   _____ Lung or breathing problems
    _____ Angina   _____ Unexplained weight loss
    _____ Irregular heartbeat   _____ Cancer of (_____)
    _____ Other heart problems   _____ Other tumor (_____)
    _____ Rheumatic fever   _____ Blood transfusions
    _____ Tuberculosis   _____ Hepatitis
    _____ Glaucoma   _____ AIDS
    _____ Multiple sclerosis   _____ Meningitis

41. Do any blood relatives have:

    _____ Diabetes   _____ Cancer

    _____ Hypoglycemia   _____ Heart disease

    _____ Other major medical problems such as those above. Please specify:

42. Describe serious accidents *unless* directly related to your doctor's visit here.

    _____ None

    _____ Occurred with head injury, loss of consciousness, or whiplash

    _____ Occurred without head injury, loss of consciousness, or whiplash
    Describe:

43. List all current medications and doses (include birth control pills and vitamins).

44. Medication allergies

    _____ None   _____ Novocaine

    _____ Penicillin   _____ Iodine

    _____ Sulfa   _____ Codeine

    _____ Tetracycline   _____ Adhesive tape

    _____ Erythromycin   _____ Aspirin

    _____ Keflex/Ceclor/Ceftin   _____ X-ray dyes

    _____ Other: (Please specify.)

45. List operations

    _____ Tonsillectomy (age _____)

    _____ Appendectomy (age _____)

    _____ Adenoidectomy (age _____)

    _____ Heart surgery (age _____)

    _____ Other: (Please specify.)

46. List toxic drugs or chemicals to which you have been exposed:

    _____ Lead

    _____ Streptomycin, neomycin, kanamycin

    _____ Mercury

    _____ Other: (Please specify.)

47. Have you had x-ray *treatments* to your head or neck (including treatments for acne or ear problems as a child, treatments for cancer, etc.)?
    Yes _____   No _____

48. Describe serious health problems of your spouse or children.

    _____ None

APPENDIX 2–3

Case History: Supplemental Form
for Paradoxical Vocal Cord Dysfunction[1]

University of Wisconsin Hospital & Clinics
Otolaryngology/Voice Clinic

NAME_____DOB_____SEX_____
MR#_____HEIGHT_____WEIGHT_____DATE_____
OCCUPATION_____

PLEASE ANSWER THE FOLLOWING QUESTIONS:

1. How long have you had your present breathing problem?

    Have you ever had other breathing problems?

    What do you think caused your present breathing problem?

    Did your breathing problem come on slowly or suddenly?

    Is it getting: Worse_____. Better_____. Same_____.

    Can you do anything that helps make it better?

    Do you have asthma? If yes, when was it diagnosed?

    Do you have allergies? If yes, to what?

2. Which of these statements best describes your breathing problems?

I can't get enough air.	Yes	No	Sometimes
I run out of air while speaking.	Yes	No	Sometimes
My chest feels tight.	Yes	No	Sometimes
My throat feels tight.	Yes	No	Sometimes
I can't coordinate my breathing with my speech	Yes	No	Sometimes
This is different than asthma.	Yes	No	Sometimes
This is the same as asthma but my inhalers don't work.	Yes	No	Sometimes
Nothing I do helps my breathing.	Yes	No	Sometimes

[1]Reprinted with permission of the University of Wisconsin Hospital and Clinics.

3. Which of these are related to your breathing difficulties?

    _____ Exercise induced
    _____ Occurs at night
    _____ Occurs while sitting
    _____ Stress induced
    _____ Co-occurs with coughing
    _____ Limits activities

4. What medications are you taking for your breathing problems?

5. Are you taking any other medications? If YES, please list meds and indicate on attached check list all that apply.

6. Have you ever had any of the following swallowing problems?

    _____ choking while eating
    _____ choking while drinking cold or hot drinks
    _____ choking while eating spicy foods
    _____ choking while sitting watching TV

7. If you choke how frequently does it occur?

8. During the PAST MONTH have you often experienced any of the following?
    _____ stomach pain
    _____ back pain
    _____ pain in your arms, legs, or joints
    _____ menstrual pain or PMS
    _____ pain or problems during sexual intercourse
    _____ headaches
    _____ chest pains
    _____ dizziness
    _____ fainting spells
    _____ feeling your heart pound or race
    _____ shortness of breath
    _____ constipation, loose bowels, or diarrhea
    _____ nausea, gas, or indigestion
    _____ bitter taste in mouth
    _____ burping
    _____ burning sensation in throat

8. *(continued)* during the PAST MONTH have you often experienced any of the following?
_____ frequently exercise (weight lifting, aerobics)
_____ frequently thirsty, dehydrated
_____ feeling tired or having low energy
_____ trouble sleeping
_____ the thought that you have a serious undiagnosed disease
_____ your eating being out of control
_____ generalized stress
_____ little interest or pleasure in doing things
_____ worrying about a lot of different things
_____ an anxiety attack
_____ problems with family, friends, co-workers, finances
_____ problems at school or work
_____ thought about cutting down on alcohol, tobacco, or drugs
_____ had more than 5 drinks in one day
_____ nausea or upset stomach
_____ live, work, or perform around smoke or fumes

9. Do you have any neurological problem (tremor, Parkinson's disease)?

10. Have you had any emotional problems that were treated by a psychologist or psychiatrist or by medication?

11. Have you had any medical problems? If YES explain.

12. Have you ever had surgery? YES NO If yes list date and type

_____
_____
_____
_____
_____
_____

13. Do you have any problems with your voice? YES   NO   (IF NO, GO ON TO QUESTION 15.)
Did your voice problem come on slowly or suddenly?

Is it getting: _____Worse   _____Better   _____Same_____

Did it begin before or after your breathing problems began?

Is it different when you have breathing problems?

14. Do you experience any of the following?
    _____ Hoarseness (coarse and scratchy sounding voice)
    _____ Fatigue (voice tires or changes quality after singing or speaking for a short period of time)
    _____ Increased effort to talk
    _____ Volume disturbance softly_____loudly_____
    _____ Loss of range (high _____low_____)
    _____ Change in classification (example: voice lowered from soprano to mezzo)
    _____ Breathiness
    _____ Voice worse in the morning
    _____ Voice worse later in the day, after it has been used
    _____ Profuse sweating
    _____ Tingling or numbness in parts of body
    _____ Afraid you were dying or had bad disease
    _____ Chest cough
    _____ Eat late at night
    _____ Clear your throat a lot
    _____ Frequent bad breath
    _____ Traveled recently: When and where
    _____ Tickling or choking sensation
    _____ Pain in throat while speaking or singing
    _____ Jaw joint problems
    _____ Bitter or acid taste, or bad breath first thing in the morning
    _____ Frequent "heartburn" or hiatal hernia
    _____ Speak extensively (e.g., teacher, clergy, attorney, telephone work)***
    _____ Sing daily, in choirs, semi-professionally or professionally
    _____ Frequently clear your throat
    _____ Frequently whisper
    _____ Frequently yell or talk loud
    _____ Work around extreme dryness

*** IF YES WE WOULD LIKE TO ASK YOU TO COMPLETE AN ADDITIONAL FORM
DESIGNED ESPECIALLY FOR PROFESSIONAL VOICE USERS.

15. Do you have, or suspect you have, any of these medical conditions? (if YES, explain).

AIDS	No_____Yes	_____
Arthritis	No_____Yes	_____
Asthma	No_____Yes	_____
Breathing problems	No_____Yes	_____
Cold	No_____Yes	_____
Diabetes	No_____Yes	_____
Digestion problems	No_____Yes	_____

Ear problems	No_____	Yes_____
Excessive sweating	No_____	Yes_____
Eye disease	No_____	Yes_____
Frequent cold sores	No_____	Yes_____
Gonorrhea	No_____	Yes_____
Hay fever	No_____	Yes_____
Hearing problems	No_____	Yes_____
Heart problems	No_____	Yes_____
Hepatitis	No_____	Yes_____
Hernia	No_____	Yes_____
Herpes infection	No_____	Yes_____
High blood pressure	No_____	Yes_____
Hormone problems	No_____	Yes_____
Kidney problems	No_____	Yes_____
Loss of hair	No_____	Yes_____
Low blood pressure	No_____	Yes_____
Lung problems	No_____	Yes_____
Muscle spasms	No_____	Yes_____
Neck problems	No_____	Yes_____
Neurological problems	No_____	Yes_____
Nose problems	No_____	Yes_____
Numbness in arms, face, legs	No_____	Yes_____
Psychiatric problems	No_____	Yes_____
Psychological problems	No_____	Yes_____
Sensitive to cold/heat/touch	No_____	Yes_____
Shaking	No_____	Yes_____
Sinus problems	No_____	Yes_____
Skin problems	No_____	Yes_____
Sleeping problems	No_____	Yes_____
Speech problems	No_____	Yes_____
Swallowing problems	No_____	Yes_____
Syphilis	No_____	Yes_____
Throat problems	No_____	Yes_____
Thyroid problems	No_____	Yes_____
Tingling in arms, face, legs	No_____	Yes_____
Tremors	No_____	Yes_____
Tuberculosis	No_____	Yes_____
Ulcers	No_____	Yes_____
Urinary problems	No_____	Yes_____
Vision problems	No_____	Yes_____
Walking problems	No_____	Yes_____

Other (please describe)_____

16. On the back of this page please list all of your current health care providers (doctors, speech pathologists, physical therapists, etc.).

APPENDIX 2–4

Spasmodic Dysphonia Study

DEMOGRAPHIC DATA AND CASE HISTORY QUESTIONNAIRE

Name: |_|_|_|_|_|_|_|_|_|_|_| |_|_|_|_|_|_|_|_|_|_|_| Medical Record No.: |_|_|_|_|_|_|_|_|
     Last   First

Social Security: |_|_|_|-|_|_|_|-|_|_|_|_| Date of Birth: |_|_|_|_|_|_|_|_| Sex: M ☐   F ☐

Address: _____   Racial Background:

City: _____ State _____   ☐ Asian

Zip: _____   ☐ Black

Telephone: (|_|_|_|) |_|_|_|-|_|_|_|_| ☐ Caucasian

    ☐ Hispanic

    ☐ Other (specify)

History

_____

1. How long have you had a voice problem? _____

2. Who noticed your voice problem first? _____

3. Did your voice problem begin gradually? .... Yes ☐   No ☐

4. If NO, did the sudden onset begin:

  a. with viral illness? .... Yes ☐   No ☐

  b. following trauma or injury? .... Yes ☐   No ☐

       Trauma type: ☐ blow to the face   ☐ blow to the head   ☐ blow to the neck

  c. following emotional trauma? .... Yes ☐   No ☐

  d. following surgery? .... Yes ☐   No ☐

      Surgery type (check all that apply):

         ☐ Thyroid   Date (s): _____

         ☐ Chest   Date (s): _____

         ☐ Endarterectomy   Date (s): _____

         ☐ Laryngeal (specify types below):

            ☐ hemilaryngectomy   Date (s): _____

            ☐ cordectomy   Date (s): _____

            ☐ focal lesion excised   Date (s): _____

            ☐ teflon injection   Type/date (s): _____

            ☐ other laryngeal surgery   Date (s): _____

        ☐ Other surgery   Specify: _____

      On a 5-point scale, please rate the effects of each prior surgery on your voice:

1 = much better;   2 = somewhat better;   3 = no change;   4 = somewhat worse;   5 = much worse.

      Surgical Procedure   one month after surgery   currently

      _____

      _____

      _____

  e. due to some cause not mentioned above? (please specify) _____

5. How does your voice today compare to your voice when the problem began?

☐ much better   ☐ somewhat worse   ☐ no change

☐ somewhat better   ☐ much worse

6. How long has your voice been at its present level of functioning? _____

7. When you are fatigued, is your voice the same, better, or worse? _____

8. Do you have difficulty communicating in noisy environments? .... Yes ☐   No ☐

9. Do you have difficulty communicating in quiet environments? .... Yes ☐   No ☐

10. Do you have difficulty being understood when you talk? .... Yes ☐   No ☐

11. Does your voice quality vary? .... Yes ☐   No ☐

12. Is your voice ever normal? .... Yes ☐   No ☐

13. For each situation given below, please enter the number that best describes your level of difficulty communicating:

|_| Moving cars |_| Talking to strangers

|_| Restaurants |_| Singing

|_| Parties |_| Unfamiliar environments

|_| Out-of-doors |_| Talking to family and friends

|_| Telephone |_| Whispering

SCALE
1 – no problem
2 – occasional problems
3 – general difficulty
4 – extreme difficulty
5 – impossible to communicate

14. Using the 5-point scale given below, please indicate how often each item listed is a problem for you.

|_| vocal fatigue |_| Choking on liquids

|_| Loudness of voice |_| Choking on solids

|_| Pitch of voice |_| Effort to talk

|_| Quality of voice |_| Ability to talk on phone

|_| Swallowing |_| Breathing

                         |_| Hearing

SCALE
1 – never a problem
2 – rarely a problem
3 – occasionally a problem
4 – frequently a problem
5 – severe disability, always a
       problem

15. Please check all answers that apply to you:

____ Voice worse in the morning

____ Voice worse later in the day, after
     it has been used

____ Have had voice training (When?)

_____

____ Speak extensively (e.g., teacher, clergy
     attorney, telephone, work, etc.)

____ Cheerleader

____ Speak extensively in noisy environments

____ Bitter or acid taste; bad breath or hoarse-
     ness first thing in the morning

____ Eat late at night

____ Eat any of the following before speaking:

     ____ chocolate   ____ milk or ice cream

     ____ coffee   ____ nuts

     ____ alcohol   ____ highly spiced food

____ Under particular stress at present

____ Live or work around smoke or other fumes

____ Live or work in a very dry or dusty area

____ Traveled recently

     Where? _____

     When? _____

16. What is your occupation? _____

17. How important is your voice in everyday activities?
    - ☐ very important—critical to my functioning, use voice a lot
    - ☐ somewhat important
    - ☐ neutral—doesn't affect activities
    - ☐ somewhat unimportant
    - ☐ very unimportant—rarely use voice

18. Has your voice had any effect on your daily activities?
    - ☐ voice has had a very positive effect on activities
    - ☐ voice has had a small positive effect on activities
    - ☐ voice has had no effect on activities
    - ☐ voice has had small negative effect on activities
    - ☐ voice has had very negative effect on activities

19. Has your voice added to life stresses? _____

    _____

    _____

    _____

20. Have you ever had voice therapy? . . . . Yes ☐ No ☐

    If YES, please give names, dates, places, and brief description of treatment. If treatment was effective indicate how long you had remission of symptoms.

Dates	Name of Speech Pathologist	Address	Type of Therapy	Effectiveness

21. Have you ever had medical treatment for your voice problem? . . . . Yes ☐ No ☐

    If YES, please give names, dates, places, and brief description of treatment. If treatment was effective indicate how long you had remission of symptoms.

Dates	Name of Physician	Address	Type of Therapy	Effectiveness

22. Your family doctor's name, address, and telephone   Your laryngologist's name, address, and telephone

    _____   _____

    _____   _____

    _____   _____

    _____   _____

23. Have you ever been evaluated by an allergist? . . . . Yes ☐   No ☐

    If YES, please give name, address, and results.

    _____

    _____

    _____

24. Have you ever consulted a psychologist or psychiatrist? . . . . Yes ☐   No ☐

25. Please list any surgeries you have not yet mentioned:
    - ☐ Tonsils (date) _____
    - ☐ Adenoids (date) _____

    Others _____

    _____

    _____

26. Have you had a cold recently? . . . . Yes ☐   No ☐

    If YES, list any symptoms that are still present:

    _____

27. Have you had x-ray therapy to your head, neck, or face? . . . . Yes ☐   No ☐

28. Have you been exposed to any of the following chemicals at home or at work?
    Check all that apply:

    ____ Carbon monoxide   ____ Arsenic

    ____ Mercury   ____ Aniline dyes

    ____ Insecticides   ____ Industrial solvents (benzene, etc.)

    ____ Lead

    ____ Other (list) _____

    _____

29. How many packs of cigarettes do you smoke per day, and for how many years? _____

30. If you used to smoke, how much did you smoke, for how many years, and when did you stop? __

    _____

31. Does your spouse or roommate smoke? . . . . Yes ☐   No ☐

32. How much alcohol do you drink? _____

33. Did you used to drink more heavily? . . . . Yes ☐   No ☐

34. How many cups of coffee, tea, cola, or other caffeine-containing drinks do you drink per day? __

    _____

35. List other drugs you use such as marijuana, cocaine, etc.: _____

36. Have you noticed any of the following? Check all that apply:

    ____ Hypersensitivity to heat or cold   ____ Blurred vision or blindness

    ____ Excessive sweating   ____ Weakness or paralysis of the face

    ____ Change in weight: ☐ gained ☐ lost   ____ Clumsiness in arms or legs

    ____ lbs in ____ weeks ____ months   ____ Confusion or loss of memory

    ____ Change in your voice   ____ Difficulty with speech

_____ Change in skin or hair   _____ Difficulty with swallowing

_____ Palpitation (fluttering) of the heart   _____ Seizure (epileptic fit)

_____ Emotional lability (swings of mood)   _____ Pain in the neck or shoulder

_____ Double vision   _____ Shaking or tremors

_____ Numbness of the face or extremities   _____ Memory change

_____ Tingling around the mouth or face   _____ Personality change

37. At what age did you reach puberty? _____

38. Do you nave any significant illness? (If YES, explain)?

     1. allergies to medicine   Yes ☐   No ☐ _____

     2. other allergies   Yes ☐   No ☐ _____

     3. arthritis   Yes ☐   No ☐ _____

     4. asthma or lung problems   Yes ☐   No ☐ _____

     5. cold sores or Herpes infections   Yes ☐   No ☐ _____

     6. diabetes   Yes ☐   No ☐ _____

     7. esophageal refluxes   Yes ☐   No ☐ _____

     8. frequent colds   Yes ☐   No ☐ _____

     9. frequent throat infections   Yes ☐   No ☐ _____

     10. gastrointestinal problems   Yes ☐   No ☐ _____

     11. hay fever   Yes ☐   No ☐ _____

     12. hearing impairment   Yes ☐   No ☐ _____

     13. heart problem   Yes ☐   No ☐ _____

     14. high blood pressure   Yes ☐   No ☐ _____

     15. hormone problem   Yes ☐   No ☐ _____

     16. kidney problems   Yes ☐   No ☐ _____

     17. liver disease   Yes ☐   No ☐ _____

     18. lung disease   Yes ☐   No ☐ _____

     19. neurological disease   Yes ☐   No ☐ _____

     20. pneumonia   Yes ☐   No ☐ _____

     21. rheumatic fever   Yes ☐   No ☐ _____

     22. sinus problems   Yes ☐   No ☐ _____

     23. syphilis or gonorrhea   Yes ☐   No ☐ _____

     24. thyroid disease   Yes ☐   No ☐ _____

     25. tuberculosis   Yes ☐   No ☐ _____

     26. ulcers   Yes ☐   No ☐ _____

     27. urinary tract infection   Yes ☐   No ☐ _____

     28. other (specify)   Yes ☐   No ☐ _____

39. Are you on any medications? (If YES, explain) _____

     1. aspirin   Yes ☐   No ☐ _____

     2. antihistamines   Yes ☐   No ☐ _____

     3. allergy pills   Yes ☐   No ☐ _____

     4. tranquilizers   Yes ☐   No ☐ _____

5. oral contraceptives	Yes ☐	No ☐ _____
6. hormone pills	Yes ☐	No ☐ _____
7. diuretics	Yes ☐	No ☐ _____
8. diet pills	Yes ☐	No ☐ _____
9. blood pressure medicines	Yes ☐	No ☐ _____
10. anti-inflammatory medicines	Yes ☐	No ☐ _____
11. mood elevators	Yes ☐	No ☐ _____
12. other (specify)	Yes ☐	No ☐ _____

40. Do you have any questions or concerns about your voice?_____

_____

_____

APPENDIX 2–5

UVP Patient History

Center: UI　UT　WI
Study ID # ___ ___ ___
Hospital # _____
Date Complete #___/___/___

1. When did you first notice that you had a voice problem?

___ ___ - ___ ___
　MO　　YR

2. When did you first see a doctor about your voice problem?

___ ___ - ___ ___
　MO　　YR

3. Who first noticed it?_____

4.　Do any of the following appear to be related to the ONSET of your voice problem? (check YES or NO for each answer)	Yes	No
personal injury		
health problem (specify _____)		
general anesthesia		
surgery		
other (specify _____)		

5.　Are any of the following related to the SEVERITY of your problem? (check YES or NO for each answer)	Yes	No
smoking		
health problem (specify _____)		
noise at work		
yelling or shouting		
diet		
work environment		
emotional stress		
speaking for extended periods of time		
recent emotional event such as loss of loved one or marital problem		
singing technique		
singing a demanding role		
other (specify _____)		

6. Has the onset of the problem been gradual or sudden?

____ gradual

____ sudden

7. Since you first noticed your voice problem, has your voice gotten:

____ better

____ same

____ worse

8. Which symptoms do you CURRENTLY have? (check YES or NO for each symptom)	Yes	No
hoarseness (coarse or scratchy sound)		
voice tires or changes quality after singing or speaking for a short period of time		
trouble speaking over noise		
trouble speaking or singing softly		
difficulty projecting voice		
loss of high range		
loss of low range		
prolonged warm-up time (over 1/2 hour to warm up voice)		
breathiness		
tickling or choking sensation while using voice		
pain in throat when using voice		
voice is worse in the morning		
voice worse later in the day, after it has been used		
frequently clear your throat		
bitter or acid taste		
bad breath in the morning		
hoarseness first thing in the morning		
laryngitis more than twice a year		
increased effort to talk		
brweathing difficulties		
swallowing difficulties		
choking sensation when not using voice		
voice strain		
other (specify _____)		

9. Have you noticed any of the following symptoms since the ONSET of your voice problem? (check YES or NO)	Yes	No
hypersensitivity to heat or cold		
excessive sweating		
weight gain (___ lbs)		
weight loss (___ lbs)		
palpitation (fluttering) of the heart		
emotional lability (swings of mood)		
double vision		
numbness of the face or extremities		
numbness elsewhere on body		
tingling around the mouth or face		
blurred vision or blindness		
weakness or paralysis of the face		
clumsiness in arms or legs		
confusion or loss of consciousness		
seizure (epilepsy)		
pain in the neck or shoulder		
memory change		
personality change		
head tremor		
other tremors or shaking		
changes in handwriting		
weakness of hand, arm, or leg		
unsteadiness		
extreme muscle fatigue		
lump in throat		

10. Do you have any medical problems? (check YES or NO to each condition)	Yes	No
high blood pressure		
heart problems		
diabetes		
arthritis, joint, or muscle pain		
hepatitis		
tuberculosis		
syphilis or gonorrhea		
HIV virus		
asthma or lung problems		
kidney problems		
neurological problems		
Parkinson's disease		
hearing problems		
psychiatric problems		
thyroid problems		
other (specify _____)		

11. List any previous operations:

Surgery	Age	Hospital/Physician

12. Are you currently being seen by a neurologist?

_____ no

_____ yes

13. Do you currently have an infection?

_____ no

_____ yes

14. For women, are you/or do you think you are pregnant?

    _____ no

    _____ yes

15. Have you been evaluated by an allergist?

    _____ no

    _____ yes

16. Are you allergic to: (check YES or NO for each drug)	Yes	No
penicillin		
sulfa		
iodine		
tetracycline		
novacaine		
other medicine (specify _____)		
food (specify _____)		
other (specify _____)		

17. Which medicine do you take currently and what is the dosage?	Yes	No	Name of Drug	Dosage
aspirin				
asthma medication				
allergy medication				
antihistamines				
anti-inflammatory				
birth control pills				
blood pressure medication				
diet pills				
decongestant				
muscle relaxants				
medicine for neurologic problems				
medicine for anxiety or depression				
other (specify _____)				

18. Have you ever smoked tobacco products?

    ____ yes

    ____ no

19. Do you currently smoke?

    ____ yes

    ____ no

20. Have you been exposed to any of the following chemicals at home or at work? (check all that apply)	Yes	No
carbon monoxide		
mercury		
insecticides		
lead		
arsenic		
aniline dyes		
industrial solvents (benzine, etc.)		
other (chemicals or fumes)		

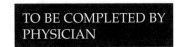

Center: UI   UT   WI
Study ID # ___ ___ ___
Hospital # _____
Date Complete #___/___/___

UVP MEDICAL FORM

Name: _____

Date of Onset _____ Age _____ Weight _____ Height _____

Presumed Etiology	YES	NO
Chest/Mediastinum/Cardiomyopathy		
CNS		
Presumed Iatrogenic		
Intubation		
RLN Severed		
Neuropathy		
Thyroid Disease		
Trauma		
Idiopathic		

Presence of	YES	NO
Abnormal Laryngeal Sensation		
Adequate Airway		
Dysphagia		
Increased Effort to Talk		
Problem with Vocal Quality		
Unilateral Vocal Fold Paralysis		
Vocal Fatigue		

_____   _____

Signature of Physician   Date

CHAPTER

THE PATIENT HISTORY

The Art of Observational Assessment

"He alone is an acute observer who can observe minutely without being observed."
—Lavater

The second component of the patient history is observational assessment. Interpersonally, observational assessment is a process of perceiving characteristics that may indicate a patient's physical status and behavioral function, without drawing unnecessary attention to the observational process that might jeopardize rapport with the patient. Professionally-technically, the process culminates in formation of a clinical impression about the significance of the observational findings, in light of other available information. Clinicians employ both art and science, using informal and formal procedures, to complete observational assessment.

INFORMAL OBSERVATIONAL ASSESSMENT

The skilled clinician connects with the patient across the spectrum of the senses. Primary to the assessment process are observations made through sight and hearing; to a lesser degree touch and smell also reveal relevant information about an individual. The clinical impressions formed during this portion of the evaluation help the clinician develop diagnostic hypotheses that will undergo further scrutiny, clarification, and refinement.

Visual Evaluation

The sense of sight is a fundamental tool that is used in evaluating five aspects of the patient's presentation:

▶ General appearance,
▶ Posture, breathing, and musculoskeletal tension,
▶ Neurological dysfunction,
▶ Physical dysmorphology,
▶ Clinical manifestations of disease.

General Appearance

In evaluating a patient's general appearance, several signs of health and well-being are surveyed. The patient's age, height and weight, facial expression, posture and ambulation, and the condition of the skin, hair, and nails are all noted. Other relevant visual evaluations of general appearance might include the individual's personal hygiene and observations of the head and neck.

Age. When making observations about the patient's age, the examiner compares chronological age to predicted age. If a patient appears to be much older than his or her chronological age, then several possible aging factors are considered such as depression, chronic illness, or an abusive lifestyle. Conversely, if a patient appears much younger and less mature than his or her chronological age, then the clinician determines if the immaturity is related to the individual's pragmatics, dress, and/or voice. Examples of voice characteristics that could contribute to the perception of immaturity include the thin high-pitched voice of the post-pubertal male who is speaking in falsetto or the weak "baby voice" of the adult female who is speaking with a high, anterior tongue carriage and generalized oral constriction. Both these conditions are typically associated with psychological immaturities or conflicts.

Height and Weight. A visual inspection of the patient's height and weight is made since weight problems (e.g., abnormal thin-

ness or obesity) or sudden changes in weight can be associated with a variety of disorders that may affect the voice. Sudden weight loss could be related to an eating disorder, gastrointestinal disease, psychological problems (e.g., depression) or other medical conditions (e.g., diffuse carinomatosis, Addison's disease, or hyperthyroidism).

Patients who are abnormally thin may have poor nutritional habits or have swallowing problems, be anorexic or bulimic or have other health problems (e.g., gastrointestinal disease). A 5 ft. 5 in., 92-lb. female voice patient, who suffered from constant nausea and vomiting because of delayed gastric emptying, found that her voice and weight problems were alleviated when a feeding tube was inserted into her stomach through a gastrostomy: the chronic vomiting was producing laryngeal irritation from both the stomach acids and from the mechanical trauma of emesis.

Obese patients might be at greater risk for developing voice and health problems related to sleep apnea, respiratory distress, adult-onset diabetes, or gastroesophageal reflux. One 5 ft. 10 in., 330-lb. male developed all of these complications, secondary to obesity.

Facial Expression. A patient's facial expression can offer useful information about the person's affective state as well as about his or her physical status. For example, clinicians might observe the vacant, fixed staring expression of the Parkinson patient; the flat and saddened look of the patient with clinically overt depression; or the very common facial postures indicating anxiety states. *A Parkinson patient taking an anti-Parkinson agent (pergolide mesylate) that has the common side effect of producing hallucinations, began seeing 3-foot-tall cats and rats. His concerned facial expression and searching looks into space were the first signs of the drug reaction.* Visible signs of physical discomfort may be observed in acutely ill patients or in those suffering chronic pain from conditions such as rheumatoid arthritis.

Posture and Ambulation. Body posture and ambulation are of concern to the voice clinician since proper voice production depends upon having a well-aligned skeletal system that can be maintained with and without physical activity. The postural and ambulatory changes that are part of the normal aging process (Figure 3–1) need to be recognized. Normal aging changes must also be differentiated from those related to neurological diseases (e.g., Parkinson's disease) and musculoskeletal diseases (e.g., rheumatoid arthritis). There is further discussion, later in this chapter, of the postural

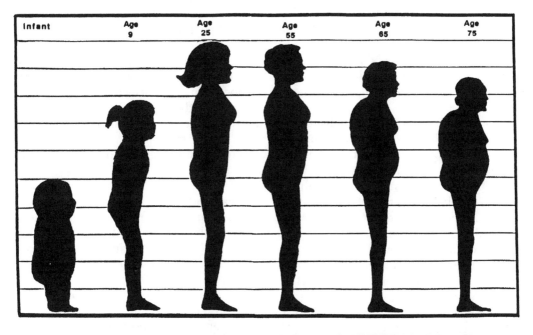

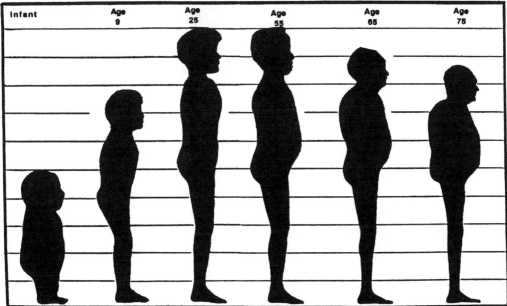

Figure 3–1. Postural changes related to the normal aging process. (Reprinted with permission from M. Hirano & D. M. Bless, 1993, p. 196. *Videostroboscopic examination of the larynx.* San Diego: Singular Publishing Group, Inc.)

changes and movement patterns that accompany selected diseases.

Skin, Hair, and Nails. Because a variety of systemic disorders manifest themselves through changes in the dermatological system, a visual screening evaluation of the patient's skin, hair, and nails is routinely made; changes in the condition of the skin, hair, and nails can be markers of internal disease. Changes in skin color or skin pigmentation are noted along with any skin rashes or skin eruptions, scaling or sloughing of the skin, and visible signs of dryness in the skin and hair.

Abnormal changes in hair distribution (e.g., excessive hair growth or hair loss or unusual hair growth patterns) or changes in hair texture (e.g., unusual coarsening or brittleness of the hair) are noteworthy as these changes may be related to a systemic condition (e.g., hypothyroidism or Cushing's syndrome) that could alter the voice.

Changes in the nails might also point to illness although nail changes can also be related to the drug therapies that are used to treat systemic dysfunctions or genetic factors. The yellow nail syndrome (i.e., diffuse yellow discoloration of the nail plate with marked reduction in nail growth rate) is an example of nail changes reflecting illness. Among the systemic disorders that have been associated with yellow nail syndrome are emphysema, sinusitis, internal malignancy of the larynx, lymphoma, sarcoma, and AIDS. Other examples of nail changes that may be significant because of their relationship to systemic conditions are clubbing of the nails (i.e., diffuse swelling of the distal digit with an increase in the angle between the nail plate and the proximal nail fold that is greater than 180°) and spooning of the nails (i.e., abnormal thinness and concavity of fingernails). Nail spooning may be a visual sign of anemia (Moschella & Hurley, 1992).

Personal Hygiene and Dress. Other signs of illness may be reflected in the patient's grooming and dress. Inattention to personal hygiene and dress is a common characteristic of persons with emotional disorders, but this can also be a sign of an organic disease (Kaplan & Sadock, 1985). One 77-year-old patient with senile dementia arrived in the voice clinic unshaven and dressed in glaringly conspicuous attire: all of his clothing, including his socks and shoes, were unmistakably mismatched. The dementia, an organic brain syndrome, had significantly impaired this patient's ability to perform even routine tasks such as shaving and dressing.

Inappropriate dress relative to the temperature and season can be an indicator of endocrinologic dysfunction. For example, patients with improperly managed hypothyroidism often have an intolerance for cold. These patients may wear excessive layers of clothing relative to the temperature or season.

Head and Neck. Several observations of the head and neck can be very informative. First of all, stains on the teeth can reveal a history of heavy smoking or coffee consumption. The presence of a nasogastric tube would suggest alimentation problems. Scars on the neck could be the sequelae of previous surgeries (e.g., tracheostomy, thyroidectomy, or phonosurgery).

All of the aforementioned visual evaluations of the patient's general appearance can assist the clinician in forming an overall impression of the individual's physical and emotional state. Other visual evaluations of factors that may relate more directly to the voice problem, also contribute important diagnostic information.

Posture, Breathing, and Musculoskeletal Tension

Postural misuses, musculoskeletal tension, and unnatural breathing patterns are behaviors that adversely influence voice production. Visual evaluation of these parameters is an integral part of the observational component of voice assessment. Scrutiny of the patient's body posture, neck region, and breathing patterns begins during the first encounter. Clinicians watch for correct or incorrect alignment of the skeletal system (i.e., alignment of the head, neck, torso, pelvis, and legs) as the patient walks from the waiting area to the interview room, as the patient sits in the examination chair, and throughout the voice evaluation. Proper skeletal alignment (Figure 3–2) allows for "natural breathing" to occur (Barlow, 1973; Lessac, 1973; Morrison & Rammage et al., 1994; Rammage, 1996). Natural breathing centers itself primarily in the abdominal area, with distention occurring simultaneously on all sides. The observation of excessive thorax and shoulder movement during breathing, rapid air intake, or noisy inspiration may be indicators of excessive muscular tension (Sataloff, 1991).

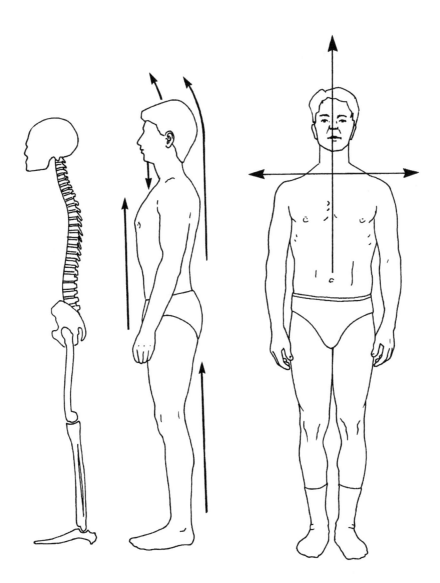

GOOD ALIGNMENT: LENGTHENING & WIDENING

Figure 3–2. Proper skeletal alignment allowing for natural speech breathing. (Reprinted with permission from M. D. Morrison & L. A. Rammage et al., 1994, p. 205. *The management of voice disorders*. London: Chapman & Hall Medical & San Diego: Singular Publishing Group.)

Physical signs of tension may also be evident at various articulatory sites. For example, jaw movements should be free and flexible, not characterized by tense, restricted posturing. Patients with temporomandibular joint disorders, dental problems (e.g., loose-fitting dentures), bruxism, or myofacial pain syndrome can develop articulatory patterns that interfere with effective voice production. Patients who "wear" a forced social smile during speech tend to exhibit restricted jaw movements as a result (Morrison & Rammage et al., 1994; Rammage, 1996).

Frequently, constellations of tension-promoting postures and behaviors may occur together, as is seen in muscular tension dysphonias (MTD). MTD, a condition commonly seen in young and middle-aged women, is manifested by excessive tension in the paralaryngeal and suprahyoid areas (Morrison et al., 1983). Morrison et al. have identified a specific cluster of physical signs that tend to characterize patients with this disorder:

▶ *"Jaw jut":* a tendency to jut the chin forward and upward;
▶ *Head retraction:* holding the atlanto-occipital and upper cervical spine areas in extension;
▶ *Larynx rise:* displacing the larynx into a position higher than neutral;
▶ *Suprahyoid tension:* hardening of the musculature underneath the chin; and
▶ *Posterior glottal chink:* triangular-shaped glottal gapping in the posterior glottis, observable during laryngeal imaging.

Assessment of the first three of these signs is performed primarily through visual observation.

Motor/Neurological Dysfunction

If a patient's motor function and gait are characterized by unsteadiness, asymmetry, rigidity, hesitation, slowness, or extraneous movements, a neurological disorder may be suspected. There are a variety of neurological problems that are associated with the dysarthrias. Dysarthrias are speech disorders resulting from disturbances in muscular control—weakness, slowness, or incoordination—of the speech mechanism due to damage to the central or peripheral nervous system or both. Such damage may affect the basic processes of respiration, phonation, resonation, articulation, and prosody (Darley, Aronson, & Brown, 1969a; 1969b; Dworkin, 1978; Yorkston, Beukelman, & Bell, 1988). Neurological disease may result in weakness and incoordination in muscle systems, including the speech mechanism, due to muscle spasticity (upper motor neuron lesions); flaccidity (lower motor neuron lesions); or other motor signs, as is characterized in the following examples:

Athetosis: Slow, writhing movements of the fingers and hands, and sometimes the toes and feet.

Cerebellar ataxia: Impaired coordination and balance, and "drunken" gait.

Chorea: Excessive motor activity, and sudden jerks and spasms of body movements.

Dystonia: Exaggerated muscle tone, resulting in inappropriate posture and incoordinate movements.

Parkinson's disease: Tremor, rigidity, bradykinesia (slowness of movement), stooped posture, shuffling of feet, and decreased arm movements.

Tremor: Slow, rhythmic fluctuations in a muscle set, causing involuntary extraneous movements at rest (resting or postural tremor); or unsteadiness and incoordination during a specific activity (action or intention tremor).

Abnormal, involuntary postures or movements may also be observed in patients who have neurological syndromes that are not always associated with a dysarthria:

Blepharospasm: Spasmodic winking, or involuntary closing of the eyelids.

Brueghel's syndrome: Slow writhing movements of the jaw and mouth (oromandibular dystonia) plus spasmodic winking or involuntary closing of the eyelids (blepharospasm).

Meige's syndrome: Slow, writhing movements of the jaw and mouth (oromandibular dystonia) plus spasmodic winking or involuntary closing of the eyelids (blepharospasm).

Spasmodic torticollis: Fixed twisting of the neck associated with muscular contracture.

Tardive dyskinesia: Tic-like movements of the tongue, the face (especially the lower half of the face), the neck and possibly the extremities (e.g., foot tapping), occurring as a side effect of the prolonged use of antipsychotic drugs.

Tic disorders also manifest themselves as observable involuntary motor behaviors (e.g. , idiotypical eye blinking, facial grimacing, or head nodding). *The Diagnostic and Statistical Manual of Mental Disorders* (DSM–IV^{TM}, 1994) defines a tic as: "a sudden, rapid, recurrent, nonrhythmic, stereotyped motor movement or vocalization." Repetitive phonic or voice tics sometimes bring patients into the voice clinic for evaluation. Gilles de la Tourette's syndrome is one type of tic disorder, thought to be neurologic, that appears in childhood or early adolescence (Shapiro & Shapiro, 1981, 1982a, 1982b). DSM–IV^{TM} (1994) provides five diagnostic criteria for Tourette's disorder (Table 3–1).

Generally, when multiple involuntary motor behaviors co-occur with a laryngeal dystonia, dyskinesia, or vocal tic, there is a common pathophysiologic mechanism. Patients with spasmodic dysphonia, for example, sometimes demonstrate dystonias in other parts of the body such as blepharospasms or torticollis, in addition to the laryngeal involvement (Blitzer & Brin, 1992).

Physical Signs of Dysmorphology

A wide variety of physical dysmorphologies may be seen in patients with congenital disorders, as well as those who have undergone head and neck surgery. Both groups of patients are at an increased risk for concomitant disorders such as speech and voice problems.

Congenital Disorders. Congenital disorders can be associated with either a specific syndrome (e.g., Down's syndrome, Cri du Chat syndrome, or Noonan syndrome) or with a nonspecific structural malformation (e.g., nonsyndromal clefting of the palate and/or lip). Because voice differences are common in those with congenital defects, clinicians should be knowledgeable of the various dysmorphologic signs (Table 3–2).

Iatrogenic Disorders. Surgically induced conditions comprise another cause of structural deviations seen among individuals with voice disorders. Disfigurements are routinely observed by professionals caring for patients who have undergone surgical treatments for head and neck cancers. Miller and Groher (1990) define several types of surgical resections (Table 3–3) that can be per-

---

TABLE 3–1. Diagnostic criteria for Tourette's disorder.

- ▶ Both multiple motor and one or more vocal tics have been present at some time, although not necessarily concurrently.

- ▶ They occur many times a day (usually in bouts) nearly every day or intermittently throughout a period of more than 1 year, and during this period there is never a tic-free period of more than 3 consecutive months.

- ▶ The disturbance causes marked distress or significant impairment in social, occupational, or other important areas of functioning.

- ▶ The onset is before age 18 years.

- ▶ The disturbance is not due to the direct physiological effects of a substance (e.g., stimulants) or a general medical condition (e.g., Huntington's disease or postviral encephalitis).

Source: Summarized from DSM-IV^{TM} (1994).

TABLE 3–2. Signs of congenital dysmorphology.

▶ Epicanthic fold of the eyes (prominent fold of the skin in the inner corner of the eyes)

▶ Hypertelorism (wide spacing of the eyes)

▶ Ears low set or rotated

▶ Unusual hair distribution (very low hairline and heavy eyebrow growth in the upper face; unusual hair whorls; hirsutism)

▶ Simian palm creases

▶ Preauricular tags or pits just anterior to the ears

▶ Curving fingers; stiff joints

▶ Webbing of feet and hands

▶ Absence of fingernails

▶ Hypotonia of all muscles

▶ Prominent lateral ridges on the palate

▶ Malproportion of the body

▶ Asymmetry, especially in the face

▶ Postnatal growth at a consistently slow pace

Source: Adapted from *Recognizable Patterns of Human Malformation: Genetic, Embryonic, and Clinical Aspects* by D. M. Smith, 1982. Philadelphia: W.B. Saunders Co.

TABLE 3–3. Oral, pharyngeal, and laryngeal resections.

A. Glossectomies (partial or complete)

B. Extensions of glossectomies (surgery may involve structures such as the tonsil, bony or soft palate, and floor of mouth)

C. Mandibular resections (commando or composite)

D. Resections of the pharynx

E. Laryngectomies (cordectomy, total)

Source: Adapted from *Medical Speech Pathology* by R. M. Miller and M. E. Groher, 1990. Rockville, MD: Aspen Publishers.

formed to treat cancers involving the oral cavity, pharynx, and larynx.

Because alterations in the structural architecture of the vocal tract can significantly impact on the voice, comprehensive evaluation must consider the contributions of both the glottic and the supraglottic structures/resonators. Abnormal configurational settings—for example, compensatory articulatory gestures secondary to glossectomy—can

influence voice quality, loudness, and pitch.

Clinical Manifestations of Disease

Sometimes the physical appearance of a patient may suggest the presence of a related illness, disease, or head and neck syndrome. The clinical manifestations of diseases associated with voice disorders might include certain physical signs (Table 3–4).

TABLE 3–4. Physical manifestations of disease and possible causes.

MANIFESTATION	CAUSE
Generalized/localized edema	Puffiness of the face, especially around the eyes, may indicate hypothyroidism (myxedema). Diffuse swelling of the hands and feet is commonly seen in patients with systemic lupus erythematous. Patches of circumscribed swelling, involving the face, lips, tongue, glottis, and extremities, can occur in association with angioneurotic edema and allergic skin disease. Bloating, especially in the face and upper torso, can be a side effect of glucocortico-steriod therapy (e.g., prednisone) in patients using an anti-inflammatory agent to treat diseases such as arthritis.
Abnormal coloration of the skin	A jaundice/yellow pigmentation of the skin is frequently seen in patients with liver disease, renal insufficiency, and in some cases of upper GI problems. An intense reddening of the skin (photosensitivity reaction) can develop in porphyria patients on exposure to ultraviolet light. A pallor or deficiency of color, especially in the face, might be a sign of anemia. A dusky, purplish cast to the face, paired with telangiectasia (fine, red lines produced by capillary dilation), is a distinctive feature of alcoholism.
Cutaneous lesions	An erythematous "butterfly" rash, on the cheeks and bridge of nose, that is exacerbated by ultraviolet light is characteristic of lupus. In rheumatoid arthritis, a transient, erythematous rash occurs sometimes prior to the onset of joint complaints. Progressive systemic sclerosis (diffuse sclerodema) can produce widespread inflammatory, vascular and fibrotic changes in the skin, resulting in a taut, leathery, and thickened appearance, with areas of depigmentation and telangiectasia.
Alopecia (hair loss)	Patchy hair loss (alopecia areata) is frequently associated with severe psychological stress. In hypothyroidism, hair may become dry and brittle and fall out. Sometimes, the outer third of the eyebrow is lost. The side effects of chemotherapy or radiation therapy may include temporary hair loss. Chemotherapy has a common complication of total alopecia (baldness). Radiotherapy may result in hair loss within the irradiated field.
Hirsuitism and virilization	In females, one cause of excessive body hair in a male distribution pattern is Cushing's disease or hyperadrenalism. Other striking features of this syndrome are moon facies, truncal obesity, a "buffalo hump," and coarsening of the voice. Other endogenous causes of hirsuitism and virilization include polycystic ovarian disease, ovarian or adrenal tumors, adrenal hyperplasia, and anorexia nervosa.
Disorders of the joints	Temporal swelling of the joints accompanies arthritis, lupus, and other inflammatory conditions. Joint deformity usually indicates a long-standing pathologic process such as rheumatoid arthritis or acromegaly.
Excessive sweating	Intolerance of heat (hyperthermia) may be a sign of hyperthyroidism. Excessive sweating is common with porphyria and acromegaly.
Hypothermia	Patients with hypothyroidism might exhibit an increased sensitivity to cold. They may dress in unseasonably heavy clothing. These symptoms may also be present in anorexic individuals.
Tremors	Most commonly, tremors indicate neurological dysfunction. Delirium tremens (DTs) can be seen in alcoholic patients during withdrawal. In hypoglycemic patients, tremors may be triggered by a release of epinephrine. In anxious patients, tremorous shaking might accompany feelings of nervousness or anxiety.
Cranial nerve involvement	Signs such as facial palsy, visual problems, vertigo, dysphagia, and tongue atrophy or fasciculations in association with voice problems may be related to a multiple cranial neuropathy. Pathogeneses may include sarcoidosis, chronic glandular tuberculosis, nasopharyngeal tumors, and Arnold-Chiari deformity.
Abnormal movements and postures	Bizarre posturing, facial grimacing, and stereotyped mannerisms (e.g., mirror gazing) are typical of schizophrenia. In tardive dyskinesia, involuntary movements tend to be localized in the lower half of the face (facial syndrome) and/or distal extremities (peripheral syndrome). Also common are rapid involuntary foot movements. In tardive Tourette's syndrome, multifocal tic behaviors (e.g., facial, shoulder, and arm tics, vocalizations, barking sounds) develop after long-term treatment or after withdrawal from neuroleptic drugs.

Case Example:
Clinical Manifestations of Disease—Porphyria

Case history: During the month of July, a 41-year-old antique dealer came to the Voice Clinic complaining of chronic vocal strain and recurrent episodes of aphonia. She described feeling a "choking" sensation when speaking that, at times, resulted in total voice loss. In addition to her voice problems, she reported intermittent problems with dysphagia and breathing. On the day of her voice evaluation, she was totally aphonic and communicated with a whisper.

Both her medical and psychological histories were complex. Medical records indicated that urine studies had revealed an overproduction of porphyrins and confirmed a diagnosis of porphyria, a metabolic disturbance related to defective enzymatic liver regulation. Her associated medical symptoms, which were classic of the disorder, included photosensitivity, recurrent abdominal pains, a creeping sensation on the skin (paresthesia), and fatigue. Given her medical symptoms, her past psychological history came as no surprise: nervousness, emotional instability, and emotional, angry outbursts are neuropsychiatric symptoms of the disorder. Predictably, she had experienced frequent mood swings, acute anxiety attacks, numerous phobias, and had demonstrated violent and bizarre behaviors on several occasions. In one instance, she had violently knocked out windows in her home for no apparent reason.

Observational assessment: Her appearance was unremarkable with the exception of a bright red, blister-like rash that extended over her face, neck, and arms. She explained that the skin lesions were related to a light sensitivity (caused by the porphyria) that tended to worsen with exposure to sunlight, especially during the summer months.

Clinical hypothesis: It was hypothesized that the patient's voice problems were related, at least in part, to the porphyria since other patients with porphyria have also manifested similar voice symptoms (Bless, Swift, & Koschkee, 1992). Based on her symptom complex, it was further hypothesized that her vocal difficulties were hyperfunctional in nature. Porphyria has been associated with both hyperfunctional voice disorders (Bless et al., 1992) and polyneuritis with a predominantly paralytic effect (Randolph & Rotter, 1992; Walter & Israel, 1974).

Instrumental evaluation: Instrumental testing included indirect laryngoscopy and videostroboscopy. Aerodynamic and acoustic testing were not undertaken because of the aphonia. The results of laryngeal imaging revealed a normal-appearing larynx. Extreme hyperfunction and laryngospasm were evident during the patient's attempts to produce phonation. No voice improvement was noted during diagnostic probe voice therapy using videoendoscopy. Overall, the patient presented a clinical profile that was consistent with a diagnosis of porphyria.

Acceptance of the clinical hypothesis: The clinical hypothesis was accepted based on the results of instrumental testing that revealed severe laryngeal hyperfunction; however, the relationship between the voice disorder and the porphyria could not be fully established. Further diagnostic voice therapy was recommended to assist in differential diagnosis, to determine the need for possible medical management, and to establish an alternative means of communication that could be implemented at times when the patient was aphonic.

There are many diagnostic problems with cases such as this in which head and neck syndromes may masquerade as psychiatric or neurologic disorders (Bless et al., 1992). Although innumerable unanswered diagnostic and treatment questions remain regarding the interplay between psychological factors and medical factors, there can be no dispute about the importance of recognizing a related medical condition and its clinical manifestations.

This discussion continues with a review of some of the auditory manifestations that can be associated with laryngeal dysfunction. Auditory evaluation involves both informal and formal assessments. In the section that follows, informal auditory evaluation is considered; the chapter concludes with a discussion of formal auditory-perceptual measures.

Informal Auditory Evaluation

Requisite in the assessment of all voice disorders is an auditory voice evaluation. Listening to the voice during speech and during laryngeal reflexes (e.g., coughing) offers clinicians valuable information that can influence decisions about diagnosis and treatment. The sense of hearing can also assist clinicians in making observations regarding a variety of typical nonspeech behaviors: dyspnea, state of secretions, temporomandibular joint dysfunction, and vocal abuse.

Dyspnea

During the personal interview, an informal auditory assessment is made of the patient's respiration. If a patient exhibits dyspnea or labored breathing, wheezing, or laryngeal stridor, a disease or disorder of the respiratory system might be present. Wheezing, a sibilant whistling sound, is commonly caused by restriction or obstruction in the peripheral airway and can be due to asthma, bronchiolitis, or other conditions involving the bronchioles. However, a variety of intrathoracic disorders, such as diffuse lung disease, can also result in wheezing.

The auditory perception of stridor implicates the larynx and can suggest involvement of the supraglottic, glottic, or subglottic areas. Stridor, which can be heard during inhalation only, during exhalation only, or during both inhalation and exhalation (biphasic stridor), can result from poor neuromuscular control, paradoxical vocal fold movements, laryngeal webbing, vocal fold paralysis, subglottic stenosis, mass lesions in the supraglottic, glottic, or subglottic areas, or various other laryngeal or tracheal anomalies. For the speech pathologist, distinguishing stridor from wheeze can assist in diagnostic decision-making. For the physician, this distinction can have life-threatening treatment implications. For example, in one case, severe laryngeal stridor was mistaken for wheezing and was attributed to an asthmatic condition, without the necessary physical and physiological evaluations. The patient was given some medication and sent home. Several weeks later, he developed severe dyspnea which necessitated an emergency tracheostomy. Examination of the larynx revealed the patient had a large cancerous supraglottic tumor.

State of Secretions

Both too little secretion (hyposalivation) and too much secretion (hypersalivation) can signal disorders. Perceptually, severe dryness of the laryngeal muscosa can result in phonation breaks or hoarseness. Dryness of the oral mucosa (xerostomia) may interfere with effective speech sound production and voice quality. It is common for dryness of the laryngeal mucosa to accompany dryness of the oral mucosa since systemic disorders (e.g., hypothyroidism) and/or the use of some medications (e.g., antihistamines) can alter the fluid balance in the mucous membranes throughout the body.

Dryness of the oral-laryngeal mucosa may be perceived through informal auditory evaluation, primarily as a "dry/raspy/thin" voice quality, with possible accompanying articulatory imprecision. If detected, several possible factors that could account for the presence of a "dry mouth" need to be considered: medication use (e.g., diuretics, tricyclic antidepressants, or other psychotropic drugs), anxiety, poor hydration, a medical condition (e.g., Sjogren's syndrome or diabetes), or radiation therapy (Sisson & Pelzer, 1990). Radiation therapy to the head and neck can produce severe dryness of the mouth and/or throat because the salivary and mucous glands that moisten the membranes are often within the radiation treatment area. The extent of the dryness problem generally depends on which glands are affected and how severely the glands have been injured.

Conversely, a "gurgly" sound to the voice (hydrophonia) is commonly heard in patients with excessive mucus in the larynx. Patients with either structurally related or neurological swallowing problems or those who experience mucus pooling and are unable to effectively clear their secretions are likely to produce hydrophonia.

Temporomandibular Joint Dysfunction

An audible clicking sound produced during jaw opening and closing may indicate temporomandibular joint (TMJ) dysfunction. The TMJ click occurs at the point where the condyle impacts against the temporal bone, through the thin, central portion of the disc. This TMJ click is just one of many symptoms that should alert the clinician to problems in the TMJ. As joint disorders progress, changes often occur in the character, position, and intensity of the joint sounds. Crepitus, a grating or cracking ("bone on bone") sound, can develop over time as the disc attachment becomes progressively thinner (Dolwick & Sanders, 1985; Hodges, 1990; Howard, 1991).

Vocal Abuses

Many behaviors associated with vocal abuse can be demonstrated during the course of an evaluation. In addition to the abusive behaviors that occur during speaking (e.g., hard glottal attacks, loud talking), non-speech abuses can emerge that may relate to the voice disorder: throat clearing, coughing, whispering, strained or explosive vocalizations (e.g., car or airplane imitations), and grunting. Observation of these behaviors is critical to the evaluation process because of the well-established relationship that exists between abusive laryngeal behavior and voice dysfunction.

Olfactory Evaluation

Although the sense of smell contributes less to the observational assessment than the visual and auditory senses, olfaction can sometimes offer valuable information to the evaluation process. For instance, olfaction can detect the scent of alcohol in a patient who has been drinking, even when he or she has adamantly denied having an alcohol problem, and has attempted to mask or conceal the smell of liquor with mouthwashes and/or fragrances. Similarly, detecting the smell of cigarette smoke on a patient who reports no longer smoking can contribute important prognostic information to the patient's history. Other distinctive smells that provide useful information to the examiner might include the burnt-rope odor of marijuana, the fetid odor that develops in patients who fail to bathe because of depression or organic brain dysfunction, or the malodorous breath that accompanies GERD, poor dental hygiene, infection, and disease.

Tactile Evaluation

Tactile evaluation should be routinely performed to aid in the detection of musculoskeletal tension (Aronson, 1990; Roy & Leeper, 1993; Morrison & Rammage et al., 1994). Palpation of the suprahyoid, laryngeal, abdominal, and temporomandibular joint areas can expose sites of chronic muscular tension and misuse. Indicators of musculoskeletal tension might include firmness in the suprahyoid and/or abdominal regions, bulging of the temporomandibular joint, elevated posturing of the larynx and hyoid bone, narrowing of the thyrohyoid space, and resistance to laryngeal displacement, either laterally or superiorly. Morrison and Rammage et al. (1994, p. 24) describe specific methodologies that can be used to identify musculoskeletal tension in each of these four regions:

Abdominal region "With the examiner's hands on the abdomen and back and then on lateral portions of the rib cage, he/she feels for evidence of the appropriate abdomen/lower rib cage distention during inspiration at rest, and preparatory to various phonatory tasks."

Oromandibular region "With the examiner's hand placed flat over the TMJ region, 'bulging' during speech or jaw depression can be felt if exaggerated or inappropriate forward movements are being made."

Suprahyoid region "By palpating the submental region just anterior to the hyoid bone, the examiner can detect inappropriate muscle activity, in the suprahyoid muscles during inspiration, which are associated with tongue retraction, and sometimes jaw extension . . . Of particular significance is persistent hypertonicity in the suprahyoids during speech and singing; increased activity during inspiration; (and) increased activity in association with pitch or loudness dynamics."

Laryngeal region "Laryngeal posture at rest and during phonation . . . can be assessed informally by palpating the thyroid notch. The vertical position of the larynx following a swallow may be used as a reference point for rest. Exaggerated excursion of the larynx during speech or singing (more than a few millimeters) is suspect, as is phonatory, posture superior to the rest position."

Aronson (1990) and Roy and Leeper (1993) present a manual assessment method that is similar to the laryngeal musculoskeletal technique of Morrison and Rammage et al. (1994), the manual laryngeal musculoskeletal tension reduction technique. This particular approach, which can be applied diagnostically in the assessment of all patients with voice disorders, and therapeutically in the treatment of patients with muscle misuse voice disorders, objectively determines the extent of elevation and the pain in response to pressure in the the larynx:

Manual musculoskeletal tension reduction technique: By encircling the larynx with the thumb and middle finger in the region of the thyrohyoid space, it (is possible to establish) whether the space (has) been narrowed by laryngeal elevation. The presence or absence of pain (can be) detected by manually palpating in the area of (the) hyoid bone and (the) thyrohyoid space bilaterally. Detection of pain in this region suggests the presence of excessive musculoskeletal tension. (Roy & Leeper, 1993, p. 248).

A more extensive examination of musculo-skeletal posture profile can be found in Lieberman's Postural Assessment for Hyperfunctional Dysphonia (Harris, Rubin, Harris, Howard & Hirson, in press; Lieberman, 1994). Since this dynamic assessment protocol requires specific intensive training to conduct properly, it is presented further in the following section, Formal Observational Assessment.

FORMAL OBSERVATIONAL ASSESSMENT

Assessment of Posture/Alignment/Muscle Misuse

Although imbalanced or inappropriate posture is readily accepted as a major factor contributing to vocal dysfunction, very few protocols for formal assessment of postural/ muscle misuse have been developed for use in voice clinics. Typical formats for informal assessment by visual observation and light palpation have been described in previous sections. The task of developing more formalized procedures and scales has been undertaken primarily in interdisciplinary clinics, particularly those with access to the expertise of practitioners of osteopathy, physical therapy, and related disciplines. The work of Harris and Lieberman (1993, 1994), and Harris et al. (in press) reflects such an interdisciplinary influence. The Lieberman Postural Assessment protocol for Hyperfunctional Dysphonia directs the clinician to specify postural misuses that fall into two primary subgroups of mechanical-postural related voice dysfunction: general posture related factors; and local laryngeal mechanical dysfunction (Appendix 3–1) (Lieberman, 1994).

> In the general posture related problems, one can talk about the effects of posture on the position of (the) larynx through the pull of the inferior and superior strap muscles, e.g., deviation of the larynx away from the midline is usually associated with rotation of the torso due to spinal scoliosis. Cervical lordosis and head position will affect the position of the larynx through the superior straps, and so on.
>
> In the local laryngeal posture, one can talk about the effects of mechanical hyperfunction on the larynx proper: . . . the Crico-Thyroid joint, Thyro-Hyoid apparatus, and internal laryngeal structures, such as arytenoid mobility, the state of the constrictor muscles, etc. . . . (realistically) in vivo, it is very difficult to separate general posture and head position from the internal laryngeal mechanics.
>
> . . . In summary, while improving posture will help voice production, not every voice problem is posture related. One needs to be specific in the assessment and diagnosis of which structures are involved. . . " (Lieberman, personal communication, September, 1996)

It is clear that in order to conduct a detailed examination of the musculo-skeletal system relating to voice function, special training and expertise is required for proper, safe procedures to be followed and for accurate interpretation of the findings.

Perceptual-Acoustic Assessment

In evaluating the psychoacoustics of voice, the clinician makes measurements of specific features such as pitch, loudness, and voice quality, using one of the scaling techniques that accommodates this type of procedure. Most commonly, equal-appearing interval scales such as the GRBAS scale (Hirano, 1981), the Buffalo III Voice Profile System (Wilson, 1987), or the Vocal Profile Analysis Scheme (Laver & MacKenzie-Beck, 1991) are used to rate phonatory and/or vocal tract dimensions. Alternative scaling procedures have been developed including the Prosody-Voice Screening Profile (Shriberg, Kwiatkowski, & Rasmussen, 1990), the M. P. Gelfer Perceptual Rating Scale (Gelfer, 1988), and the Darley, Aronson, and Brown dysarthria classification system (Darley, Aronson, & Brown, 1969). Both the Prosody-Voice Screening Profile and the dysarthria classification system use checklist scoring to generate a profile of behavior and performance.

Several groups of clinical investigators have applied Osgood's principle of semantic differentials (Osgood, Suci, & Tannenbaum, 1957) and factor analysis to generate clinically relevant terms for perceptual-acoustic assessment (Askenfelt & Hammarberg, 1986; Gelfer, 1988; Hammarberg, Fritzell, Gauffin, Sundberg, & Wedin, 1980; Isshiki, 1966; Isshiki, Okamura, Tanabe, & Morimoto, 1969; Isshiki & Takeuchi, 1970). Gelfer's protocol, originally designed for use with normal speakers, uses graded scales with semantically opposite terms at either pole (e.g., high pitch to low pitch; loud voice to soft voice; and melodious quality to raspy quality). The protocol has been adapted for use in the clinical setting (Table 3–5). In adapting the protocol, Gelfer reduced the number of semantic bipolar items, since clinical voice description requires less subtlety than does differentiation of normal voices (Pausewang Gelfer, personal communication, June 1996). For clinical use, Gelfer applies the principle of "triangulation" by providing taped samples of two "reference voices" for each bipolar item, to help listeners locate a "perceptual point" that describes a disordered voice. For example, a listener could compare a clinical voice to standard reference voices representing "high voice" and "low voice" at the ex-

TABLE 3–5. Bipolar acoustic-perceptual scales for clinical evaluation.

HIGH PITCH __ 1 __ 2 __ 3 __ 4 __ 5 __ 6 __ 7 __ 8 __ 9 __ LOW PITCH

LOUD __ 1 __ 2 __ 3 __ 4 __ 5 __ 6 __ 7 __ 8 __ 9 __ SOFT

STRONG __ 1 __ 2 __ 3 __ 4 __ 5 __ 6 __ 7 __ 8 __ 9 __ WEAK

SMOOTH __ 1 __ 2 __ 3 __ 4 __ 5 __ 6 __ 7 __ 8 __ 9 __ ROUGH

UNFORCED __ 1 __ 2 __ 3 __ 4 __ 5 __ 6 __ 7 __ 8 __ 9 __ STRAINED

BREATHY VOICE __ 1 __ 2 __ 3 __ 4 __ 5 __ 6 __ 7 __ 8 __ 9 __ FULL VOICE

HYPERNASAL __ 1 __ 2 __ 3 __ 4 __ 5 __ 6 __ 7 __ 8 __ 9 __ DENASAL

ANIMATED __ 1 __ 2 __ 3 __ 4 __ 5 __ 6 __ 7 __ 8 __ 9 __ MONOTONOUS

STEADY __ 1 __ 2 __ 3 __ 4 __ 5 __ 6 __ 7 __ 8 __ 9 __ SHAKY

SLOW RATE __ 1 __ 2 __ 3 __ 4 __ 5 __ 6 __ 7 __ 8 __ 9 __ RAPID RATE

Source: Pausewang Gelfer, Mary Lou, personal communication, June 27, 1996.

tremes of the "normal" pitch continuum, and identify a perceptual distance between the normal referents and the clinical voice. This approach provides the clinician with a tool that is dynamic: it reflects changes in the clinical voice relative to the respective normal referents. In addition to the semantic differential scale, Gelfer's clinical perceptual-acoustic protocol also includes identification of commonly recognized features of dysphonic voices: transient characteristics of pitch breaks; phonation breaks; hard glottal attacks; diplophonia; and the more constant voice quality features of breathiness; harshness and hoarseness (Pausewang Gelfer, personal communication, June 1996).

Regardless of which scaling method is used, efforts should be made to ensure reliability of ratings through adequate listener training and a thorough explanation of the basic concepts behind the scaling system. Furthermore, the validity of individual rating scales should be tested through correlational studies that examine the relationship between the listener's psychoacoustic impressions and objective, instrumental measures. To date, few psychoacoustic rating scales have met all of these criteria. Some of the available systems provide listener training tapes and user manuals (e.g., Prosody-Voice Screening Profile, Vocal Profile

Analysis), but most of the scaling systems have questionable test validity. Two scaling methods whose terms have been operationally defined in relation to test item validity (i.e., through correlational studies with instrumental measures) are the GRBAS scale and the Vocal Profile Analysis system.

GRBAS Scale

The GRBAS scale, a 4-point, equal-appearing interval scale, was proposed by the Committee for Phonatory Function of the Japanese Society of Logopedics and Phoniatrics to be used for the psychoacoustic evaluation of hoarseness (described in Hirano, 1981). This perceptually based assessment device evaluates five dimensions of deviant quality: Grade, Roughness, Breathiness, Asthenia, and Strain (Table 3–6). For each dimension, a score from 0 to 3 is used, where "0" represents nonhoarse or normal voice and "3" represents extreme severity. Together these individual ratings combine to form a profile of the patient's voice quality. For example, typical ratings for a patient with unilateral vocal fold paralysis, in the early stage of recovery, might be: $G_3 R_1 B_3 A_3 S_1$.

The GRBAS system evolved from a series of studies on the perceptual evaluation of hoarseness. Isshiki and his colleagues derived an initial set of terms using Osgood's

TABLE 3–6. Operational definitions for GRBAS dimensions.

Dimension	Characteristics
GRADE (G) Overall severity or abnormality of the dysphonia	No single acoustic measure correlates with the grade of a dysphonia.
ROUGHNESS (R) The psychoacoustic impression of irregular vocal fold vibration	Acoustically, roughness of the voice is represented by fluctuations in fundamental frequency and/or the amplitude of the glottal source spectrum. Laryngeal pathologies with associated edema and/or vocal fold asymmetry (e.g., polyps, cysts, unilateral scarring) are likely to produce a rough-sounding voice.
BREATHINESS (B) The psychoacoustic impression of air leakage through the glottis	Acoustically, the presence of white noise characterizes the perception of breathiness. Glottal openings due to vocal fold paralysis, muscle tension dysphonias, or vocal fold bowing can result in a breathy component to voice quality.
ASTHENIA (A) The psychoacoustic impression of weak voice	Acoustically, the asthenic voice lacks higher harmonics and shows instability in fundamental frequency and/or amplitude of the acoustic waveform. Voice produced with thinned vocal folds due either to an altered structure (e.g., atrophied folds) or altered function (e.g., mutational falsetto) often sounds asthenic. Reduced tension in the glottis (e.g., a sequela to closed-head injury or myasthenia gravis) can produce a similar psychoacoustic effect.
STRAIN (S) The psychoacoustic impression of effort and hyperfunction	Acoustically, strain in the voice is represented by excessive noise and/or harmonics in the high-frequency bands and an elevated fundamental frequency. Vocal pathologies produced by hyperfunctional compression of the glottic and supraglottic structures (e.g., hyperfunctional dysphonia, adductor spasmodic dysphonia) are characterized by vocal strain. Stiffness of the vibrating structure, resulting from cancer or surgery, tends to be accompanied by a significant degree of strain.

concept of semantic differentials and factor analysis (Isshiki, 1966; Isshiki, Okamura, Tanabe & Morimoto, 1969; Isshiki & Takeuchi, 1970), and subsequent investigations focused on the spectral-acoustic correlates for perceptually salient terms (Hiroto, 1967; Takahashi & Koike, 1976; Yoshida, 1979). The GRBAS items have been described and differentiated based on their spectral-acoustic correlates (Hirano, 1981) and have been used in clinical studies in conjunction with instrumental measures to describe various vocal pathologies (Hirano, Hibi, Tera-sawa, & Fujiu, 1986; Imaizumi, 1986; Takehashi et al., 1974)

Vocal Profile Analysis

The Vocal Profile Analysis (VPA) system, developed by John Laver and Janet MacKenzie-Beck at the University of Edinburgh, was designed to describe vocal tract features in both normal and pathologic speakers (Laver & MacKenzie-Beck, 1991). This sophisticated perceptual scheme, which considers the whole vocal tract, not just phonatory characteristics, is based on the concept that the lips, jaw, and tongue can contribute as much to voice quality as the larynx or the velopharyngeal system. Consequently, the VPA protocol includes judgments regarding laryngeal carriage, laryngeal tension, vocal tract tension, velopharyngeal function, phonation type, and labial, mandibular, and lingual posturing. In total, more than 20 perceptual dimensions are evaluated (Figure 3–3). Because scoring the VPA is quite complex, it cannot be used reliably without specialized training. For this purpose, intensive 4-day courses are offered on the theory and practice of the Vocal Profile Analysis system which include training in both perception and production skills.

In scoring the VPA, listeners are first asked to decide whether a neutral (baseline) or non-neutral setting has been used for each vocal tract feature. For non-neutral items, a second pass or listen is required to grade the degree of severity, either with a qualitative distinction (moderate vs. severe) or on a 6-point equal-appearing interval scale, depending on results of reliability and validity tests by the authors for a particular item. For speech pathologists, learning to differentiate "neutral" from "normal" can be one of the most challenging aspects of the VPA scoring sytem, since speech clinicians have been traditionally trained to think in terms of normal versus pathological. However,

this distinction is critical to accurate VPA scoring and must be mastered to meet reliability standards.

When completed, the VPA protocol provides a comprehensive profile of an individual's vocal quality profile. The system accommodates the subtle differences found in voice production characteristics. The identification of subtle production patterns can be appreciated when the professional voice user seeks a voice evaluation, not because of a pathological condition, but rather because of a technical voice use problem (e.g., pharyngeal constriction, tongue backing, and/or larynx rise). In other cases where a laryngeal pathology or condition has been identified (e.g., vocal nodules), important production features that may contribute to the development of the nodules can be detected perceptually: for example, a backed tongue posture and raised larynx position may be indicative of muscle misuses that contribute to hyperkinetic function during phonation and subsequent nodule formation (Morrison et al., 1983).

Several key relationships between subjective VPA ratings and objective acoustic measures have been documented by the authors. In their training materials, they include a series of key sentence spectrograms that distinguish the acoustic differences among the various articulatory and phonatory settings.

Case Example: Vocal Profile Analysis/Vocal Tract Shortening, Tension, and Constriction:

Case History: This 39-year-old, 5 ft 1 in, 110-lb female minister came to the Voice Clinic complaining of chronic vocal fatigue, inadequate volume, and pain in the neck lateral to the larynx after speaking. She stated that these symptoms had been present to some degree throughout her 10-year pastoral career. Within the previous few months, however, increased vocal difficulties had forced her to assign a number of her regular duties and responsibilities to the assistant pastor. Although she agreed that this shift in responsibilities had actually made her workload more manageable, she felt that her career was being jeopardized by her voice problems.

(continued)

Observational assessment: To assess the auditory-perceptual characteristics of this patient's speaking voice, the VPA was used to generate a profile of vocal-tract functioning (Figure 3–4). The results revealed a combination of articulatory and phonatory settings that were serving to produce a shortened and constricted vocal tract and generalized vocal tension. Specifically, several features—raised larynx, pharyngeal constriction, close jaw, restricted jaw movements, tense vocal tract, tense larynx, denasality, high mean pitch, harsh phonation type, and backed tongue body—were judged to be non-neutral.

A manual musculoskeletal tension evaluation revealed elevated posturing of the patient's larynx when speaking, and extremely hypertonic suprahyoid musculature during inspiration and speech. In addition, the patient felt pain in response to digital pressure in the region of the thyrohyoid space and masticator muscles. The manual musculoskeletal tension evaluation was supplemented by visual observations of head-retraction and jaw-jut, an elevated and immobile larynx during speech, and signs of tension in the patient's face, particularly around the eyes and jaw. These observational findings suggested that musculoskeletal tension was contributing significantly to the voice disorder.

Clinical hypothesis: It was hypothesized that the patient's voice problems were related to a musculoskeletal tension disorder.

Instrumental evaluation: Instrumental testing included laryngeal imaging as well as aerodynamic and acoustic evaluations. Spectrographic analysis, a component of the acoustic testing, was performed to assess the resonatory characteristics of the vocal tract.

Instrumental measures were consistent with the subjective voice ratings. Videostroboscopy revealed a normal structural appearance, but laryngeal rise was noted on all phonatory tasks, and a long closed phase was noted during phonation in modal register. Spectrographic analysis further confirmed the overall pattern of vocal tract tension. Acoustically, there was minimal absorption of the high frequencies (by the vocal tract walls) and sharp formant peaks.

Acceptance of the clinical hypothesis: The clinical hypothesis was accepted. Based on the VPA profile and related clinical observations, a voice therapy program was developed to promote more natural head and neck alignment, neutral jaw and tongue postures, and generalized laxness and elongation of the vocal tract. After 10 therapy sessions, a second VPA was generated; results documented significant psychoacoustic changes in voice.

As this case study exemplifies, observational assessment can aid in the diagnostic process, can assist in planning behavioral voice therapy, and can document perceptual changes in voice following treatment programs. In addition, these informal and formal observational measures can lead the clinician to a clinical hypothesis regarding the present-ing disorder. That hypothesis must subsequently be tested by instrumental analysis.

REFERENCES

Aronson, A. E. (1990). *Clinical voice disorders* (3rd ed.). New York: Thieme Stratton.

Vocal Profile Analysis Protocol

Speaker: ....   Sex: ....   Age: ....   Date of Analysis: ....   Tape: ....   Judge: ....

VOCAL TRACT FEATURES	FIRST PASS			SECOND PASS			
	Neutral	Non-neutral		SETTING	Scalar Degree		
		Moderate	Extreme		Moderate	Extreme	
					1 2 3	4 5 6	
1. Labial Features				Lip Rounding/Protrusion			
				Lip Spreading			
				Labiodentalization			
				Extensive Range			
				Minimized Range			
2. Mandibular Features				Close Jaw			
				Open Jaw			
				Protruded Jaw			
				Extensive Range			
				Minimized Range			
3. Lingual Tip/Blade Features				Advanced Tip/Blade			
				Retracted Tip/Blade			
4. Lingual Body Features				Fronted Tongue Body			
				Backed Tongue Body			
				Raised Tongue Body			
				Lowered Tongue Body			
				Extensive Range			
				Minimized Range			
5. Velopharyngeal Features				Nasal			
				Audible Nasal Escape			

LARYNGEAL FEATURES	FIRST PASS			SECOND PASS			
	Neutral	Non-neutral		SETTING	Scalar Degree		
		Moderate	Extreme		Moderate	Extreme	
					1 2 3	4 5 6	
6. Phonation Type Features				Modal voice			
				Falsetto			
				Creak(y)			
				Whisper(y)			
				Harsh			
7. Larynx Position Features				Raised Larynx			
				Lowered Larynx			

OVERALL MUSCULAR TENSION FEATURES	FIRST PASS			SECOND PASS			
	Neutral	Non-neutral		SETTING	Scalar Degree		
		Moderate	Extreme		Moderate	Extreme	
					1 2 3	4 5 6	
8. Vocal Tract Tension Features				Tense Vocal Tract			
				Lax Vocal Tract			
9. Laryngeal Tension Features				Tense Larynx			
				Lax Larynx			

Profiles of Speech Disorders' Project, Medical Research Council Grant G978/1192

Speaker: ....   Sex: ....   Age: ....   Date of Analysis: ....   Tape: ....   Judge: ....

PROSODIC FEATURES	SETTING	Scalar Degrees		
		Neutral	Moderate	Extreme
1. Pitch Features	High Mean			
	Low Mean			
	Wide Range			
	Narrow Range			
	High Variability			
	Low Variability			
2. Loudness Features	High Mean			
	Low Mean			
	Wide Range			
	Narrow Range			
	High Variability			
	Low Variability			
3. Consistency	Tremor			
TEMPORAL FEATURES				
4. Continuity	Interrupted			
5. Tempo	Fast			
	Slow			
OTHER FEATURES				
6. Denasality				
7. Pharyngeal	Constriction			

OTHER COMMENTS :

Respiratory support :   Adequate   Inadequate

Diplophonia :   Present   Absent

Profiles of Speech Disorders' Project, Medical Research Council Grant G978/1192

Figure 3–3. Vocal Profiles Analysis form. (Reprinted courtesy of J. Laver and J. MacKenzie-Beck, 1991. Margaret College, University of Edinburgh, Scotland.)

Vocal Profile Analysis Protocol

Speaker: **Patient X**   Sex: **♀**   Age: **39**   Date of Analysis: **01/06/93**   Tape: **12**   Judge: **D.K.**

VOCAL TRACT FEATURES	FIRST PASS — Neutral	Non-neutral Moderate	Non-neutral Extreme	SETTING	Scalar Degree 1	2	3	4	5	6 (Moderate/Extreme)
1. Labial Features	✓			Lip Rounding/Protrusion						
				Lip Spreading						
				Labiodentalization						
	✓			Extensive Range						
				Minimized Range						
2. Mandibular Features			✓	Close Jaw	✓					
				Open Jaw						
				Protruded Jaw						
			✓	Extensive Range						
				Minimized Range		✓				
3. Lingual Tip/Blade Features				Advanced Tip/Blade						
				Retracted Tip/Blade						
4. Lingual Body Features			✓	Fronted Tongue Body						
				Backed Tongue Body	✓					
				Raised Tongue Body						
				Lowered Tongue Body						
	✓			Extensive Range						
				Minimized Range						
5. Velopharyngeal Features	✓			Nasal						
				Audible Nasal Escape	▨					

LARYNGEAL FEATURES	FIRST PASS — Neutral	Non-neutral Moderate	Non-neutral Extreme	SETTING	Scalar Degree 1	2	3	4	5	6 (Moderate/Extreme)
6. Phonation Type Features				Modal voice						
				Falsetto						
				Creak(y)						
				Whisper(y)						
		✓		Harsh				✓		
7. Larynx Position Features		✓		Raised Larynx						✓
				Lowered Larynx						

OVERALL MUSCULAR TENSION FEATURES	FIRST PASS — Neutral	Non-neutral Moderate	Non-neutral Extreme	SETTING	Scalar Degree 1	2	3	4	5	6 (Moderate/Extreme)
8. Vocal Tract Tension Features		✓		Tense Vocal Tract	✓					
				Lax Vocal Tract						
9. Laryngeal Tension Features		✓		Tense Larynx		✓				
				Lax Larynx						

al Profiles of Speech Disorders' Project, Medical Research Council Grant G978/1192   © University of Edinburgh 1991

Speaker: **Patient X**   Sex: **♀**   Age: **39**   Date of Analysis: **01/06/93**   Tape: **12**   Judge: **D.K.**

PROSODIC FEATURES	SETTING	Scalar Degrees — Neutral	Moderate	Extreme
1. Pitch Features	High Mean		✓	
	Low Mean	✓		
	Wide Range	✓		
	Narrow Range	✓		
	High Variability	✓		
	Low Variability	✓		
2. Loudness Features	High Mean	✓		
	Low Mean	✓		
	Wide Range	✓		
	Narrow Range	✓		
	High Variability	✓		
	Low Variability	✓		
3. Consistency	Tremor	✓		
TEMPORAL FEATURES				
4. Continuity	Interrupted	✓		
5. Tempo	Fast	✓		
	Slow	✓		
OTHER FEATURES				
6. Denasality			✓	
7. Pharyngeal	Constriction		✓	

OTHER COMMENTS :

Respiratory support :   Adequate   Inadequate

Diplophonia :   Present   Absent

Profiles of Speech Disorders' Project, Medical Research Council Grant G978/1192   © University of Edinburgh 1991

Figure 3–4. VPA profile for Patient X, exhibiting vocal tract shortening, tension and constriction.

Askenfelt, A. G., & Hammarberg, B. (1986). Speech waveform perturbation analysis: A perceptual-acoustical comparison of seven measures. *Journal of Speech and Hearing Research, 29,* 50–64.

Barlow, W. (1973). *The Alexander technique.* New York: Warner Books.

Bless, D. M., Swift, E. W., & Koschkee, D. C. (1992, November). *Manifestations of voice problems in head and neck syndromes.* Miniseminar presented at the American Speech-Language-Hearing Association Annual Convention, San Antonio, TX.

Blitzer, A., & Brin, M. F. (1992). Treatment of spasmodic dysphonia (laryngeal dystonia) with local injections of botulinum toxin. *Journal of Voice, 6*(4), 356–369.

Braunwald, E., Isselbacher, K. J., Petersdorf, R. G., Wilson, J. D., Martin, J. B., & Fauci, A. S. (1987). *Harrison's principles of internal medicine* (11th ed.). New York: McGraw-Hill.

Darley, F. L., Aronson, A. E., & Brown, J. R. (1969a). Differential diagnostic patterns of dysarthria. *Journal of Speech and Hearing Research, 12,* 246–269.

Darley, F. L., Aronson, A. E., & Brown, J. R. (1969b). Clusters of deviant speech dimensions in the dysarthrias. *Journal of Speech and Hearing Research, 12,* 462–496.

Diagnostic and statistical manual of mental disorders (4th ed.) (DSM-IV™). (1994). Washington, DC American Psychiatric Association.

Dolwick, M. F., & Sanders, B. (1985). *Surgical atlas: Temporomandibular joint internal derangements and arthrosis.* St. Louis: C. V. Mosby.

Dworkin, J. P. (1978, December). A review of motor speech disorders. *Journal of National Student Speech and Hearing Association.*

Gelfer, M. P. (1988). Perceptual attributes of voice: Development and use of rating scales. *Journal of Voice, 2*(4), 320–326.

Hammarberg, B., Fritzell, J., Gauffin, J., Sundberg, J., & Wedin, L. (1980). Perceptual and acoustic correlates of abnormal voice qualities. *Acta Otolaryngologica, 90,* 441–451.

Harris, T., & Lieberman, J. (1993). The cricothyroid mechanism, its relation to vocal fatigue and vocal dysfunction. *Voice, 2,* 89–96.

Harris, T., Rubin, J., Harris, S., Howard, D., & Hirson, A. (in press). *The voice clinic handbook.* London: Whurr.

Hirano, M. (1979). Physical and anatomical studies of the structure of the vocal folds in normal and pathological states. *Proceedings of the NIH Conference on the Assessment of Vocal Pathology.*

Hirano, M. (1981). *Clinical examination of voice.* Wien/New York: Springer-Verlag.

Hirano, M., Hibi, S., Terasawa, R., & Fujiu, M. (1986). Relationship between aerodynamic, vibratory, acoustic and psychoacoustic correlates in dysphonia. *Journal of Phonetics, 14,* 445–456.

Hiroto, I. (1967). Hoarseness. Viewpoints of voice physiology. *Japanese Journal of Logopedics and Phoniatrics, 8,* 9–15.

Hodges, J. M. (1990). Managing temporomandibular joint syndrome. *Laryngoscope, 100,* 60–66.

Howard, J. (1991). Temporomandibular joint disorders, facial pain, and dental problems in performing artists. In R. T. Sataloff, A. G. Brandfonbrener, & R. J. Lederman (Eds.) *Textbook of performing arts medicine* (pp. 111–169). New York: Raven Press.

lmaizumi, S. (1986). Acoustic measures of roughness in pathological voice. *Journal of Phonetics, 14,* 457–462.

Isshiki, N. (1966). Classification of hoarseness. *Japanese Journal of Logopedics and Phoniatrics, 7,* 15–21.

Isshiki, N., Okamura, H., Tanabe, M., & Morimoto, M. (1969). Differential diagnosis of hoarseness. *Folia Phoniatrica, 21,* 9–19.

Isshiki, N., & Takeuchi, Y. (1970). Factor analysis of hoarseness. *Studia Phonologica, 5,* 37–44.

Kaplan, H. I., & Sadock, B. J. (1985). *Comprehensive textbook of psychiatry IV.* Baltimore, MD: Williams & Wilkins.

Laver, J., & MacKenzie-Beck, J. (1991). *Vocal Profile Analysis.* University of Edinburgh: Queen Margaret College.

Laver, J., & MacKenzie-Beck, J. (1992, July). *Vocal Profile Analysis course,* University of Wisconsin, Madison, WI.

Lessac, A. (1973). *The use and training of the human voice.* New York: Drama Book Publishers.

Lieberman, J. (1994). *Lieberman Postural Assessment for Hyperfunctional Dysphonia.* Sidcup, Kent: Queen Mary's Hospital Voice Disorder Research Laboratory.

Miller, R. M., & Groher, M. E. (1990). *Medical speech pathology.* Rockville, MD: Aspen Publishers.

Morrison, M., Rammage, L., Belisle, G., Pullan, B., & Nichol, H. (1983). Muscular tension dysphonia. *Journal of Otolaryngology, 12*(5), 302–306.

Morrison, M., & Rammage, L., with: Nichol, H., Pullan, B., May, P., & Salkeld, L. (1994). *The management of voice disorders.* London: Chapman & Hall Medical & San Diego: Singular Publishing Group, Inc.

Moschella, S. L., & Hurley, H. J. (1992). *Dermatology.* Philadelphia: W. B. Saunders Co.

Osgood, C. E., Suci, G. J., & Tannenbaum, P. H. (1957). *The measurement of meaning.* Urbana: University of Illinois Press.

Rammage, L. (1996). *Vocalizing with ease: A self-improvement guide.* Vancouver: Author.

Randolph, L. M., & Rotter, J. I. (1992). Hereditary disorders of the gut and liver. In W. N. Kelley (Ed). *Textbook of internal medicine* (2nd ed.). Philadelphia: J. B. Lippincott Co.

Roy, N., & Leeper, H. A. (1993). Effects of manual laryngeal musculoskeletal tension reduction technique as a treatment for functional voice disorders; Perceptual and acoustic measures. *Journal of Voice, 7*(3), 242–249.

Sataloff, R. T. (1997). *Professional voice: The science and art of clinical care.* (2nd ed.). San Diego: Singular Publishing Group.

Shapiro, A. K. & Shapiro, E. (1981). The treatment and etiology of tics and Tourette syndrome. *Comprehensive Psychiatry, 22(2),* 193–205.

Shapiro, A. K., & Shapiro, E. (1982). Tourette syndrome: History and present status. *Advances in Neurology, 35,* 17–23.

Shapiro, A. K., & Shapiro, E. (1982). An update on Tourette syndrome. *American Journal of Psychotherapy, 36*(3), 379–390.

Shriberg, L. D., Kwiatkowski, J., & Rasmussen, C. (1990). *Prosody-Voice Screening Profile.* Tucson, AZ: Communication Skill Builders.

Sisson, G. A. & Pelzer, H. J. (1990). Staging system by sites. Problems and refinements. *Otolaryngologic Clinics of North America, 18*(3), 397–402.

Smith, D. W., with contributions by Jones, K. L. (1982). *Recognizable patterns of human malformation: Genetic, embryologic, and clinical aspects.* Philadelphia: W. B. Saunders Co.

Takehashi, H., & Koike, Y. (1976). Some perceptual dimensions and acoustical correlates of pathologic voices. *Acta Otolaryngologica, 338,* 1–24.

Takehashi, H., Yoshida, M., Oshima, T., Sakamoto, K., Tsumura, S., & Yamazaki, T. (1974). On the differential diagnosis of laryngeal pathologies through the perceptual impression of the voices. *Practica Otolaryngolica (Kyoto), 67,* 1377–1385.

Walter, J. B., & Israel, M. S. (1974). *General pathology* (4th ed.). Edinburgh/London: Churchill Livingstone.

Wilson, D. K. (1987). *Voice problems of children* (3rd ed.). Baltimore: Williams & Wilkins.

Yorkston, K. M., Beukelman, D. R., & Bell, K. R. (1988). *Clinical management of dysarthric speakers.* Boston/Toronto: College-Hill Press, Little, Brown.

Yoshida, M. (1979). Study on perceptive and acoustical classification of pathological voices. *Practica Otolaryngologica (Kyoto), 72,* 249–287.

APPENDIX 3–I

LIEBERMAN POSTURAL ASSESSMENT FOR HYPERFUNCTIONAL DYSPHONIA[1]

This protocol is intended to accompanying the instructional course on the interdisciplinary assessment and treatment of hyperfunctional voice disorder in order to achieve satisfactory practitioner agreement

Tick positive findings only in the shaded boxes. Rate by single mark on analogue scale where indicated

Accurate assessment of the laryngeal musculature and cricothyroid joints is considered essential

General Considerations   I. Observation

A. Observations while the patient is sitting and giving the history of the problem, etc.

Sitting			
	Is the anterior neck compartment smooth or are the muscles very conspicuous?	Smooth	Conspicuous
	Is activity in the anterior neck compartment visible? (e.g., Obvious Omohyoid activity)	Yes?	
	Habitual head tilting?	Left	Right
	Habitual head gestures (e.g., 'yes' or 'no' by nodding)	Yes?	

B. Observations when the patient has been asked to stand passively.
    Frontal and lateral viewing required.

Standing				
	Knee Locking	Left	Right	Both
	Weight Distribution	Left	Right	Central
	Pelvic Rotation	Forwards		
	Raised shoulders (rest)	Left	Right	Both
	Weight Bearing (Center of Gravity)	Posterior Anterior • ├————————┤		

[1]Reprinted with permission of Jacob Lieberman. Copyright 1994 Queen Mary's Hospital Voice Disorder Research Laboratory.

General Considerations 2. Palpation

Palpate	Pelvic Tilt	Left	Right	
	Lumbar Spine Lordosis	Exaggerated		
	Lumbar Spine Scoliosis	Left	Right	
	Anterior Head Translocation	A. Normal posture	1-2 cms	≥3 cms
		B. Occipital contact with vertical surface without chin raising	Contact Yes?	
	Thoracic/Cervical Spine	Contact of C7 with vertical surface?		
(Osteopathic) requires the patient to lie down	Thoracic Spine Fixed Segment	Indicate level. Vertebrae		

Cervical & Laryngeal Considerations   3. Palpation

Neck Vertebrae	Cervico-dorsal vertebral shelf (Level of hyperlordotic segment)	C3-4	C5-6	Other
Posterior Musculature	Muscular tenderness lateral to shelf	Left	Right	Both
	Occipital/Submastoid tenderness (delete if N/A)	Left	Right	Both
Anterior Musculature	Sternomastoid muscles while standing erect	Lax ←———→ Hyperactive L •├———————┤ R •├———————┤		
	Suprahyoid tension	Slight ←———→ Great •├———————┤		
	Larynx in midline	Left of m/line	Right of m/line	
	Infralaryngeal strap ms.	Hyperactive	Underactive or absent	
Laryngeal Musculature	Overall tension of laryngeal suspensory muscles	Tightly held Loosely held •├———————┤		
	Possible to palpitate structures medial to the posterior margins of the Thyroid Laminae?	Left	Right	Neither
	Thyrohyoid Membranes held/reduced in area	Left	Right	Both
	Tender/guarded cricothyroid muscles	Left	Right	Both
Cricothyroid Joints	Cricoid arch position (When visor is closed)	Neutral Anterior translocation •├———————┤		
If arch is Translocated	Does it change: A. On full head flexion B. On full head extension	More so Same Less so •├———————┤ •├———————┤		
	Individual joint laxity	Greater on Left Greater on Right •├———————┤		
Visor Position	Position at rest	Widely open Neutral Closed •├———————┤		

Cervical & Laryngeal Considerations   4. Palpation of Patient Maneuvers

Ask the patient to "siren" up and down through their entire vocal range	Palpation of the C-T visor shows:	No Movement Excellent Range		
	From its "rest" position, the visor:	Opens	Closes	Both
Ask the patient to swallow twice. During the swallow, is there	Head extension?	Yes		
	Can the patient raise the larynx freely?	Yes		
	Decrease in any anterior position of cricoid arch?	Yes		

CHAPTER

INSTRUMENTAL ANALYSES

Working From A Clinical Hypothesis

Within the maze of procedures that lead to diagnosis are various instrumental tests used to assess respiratory, phonatory, resonatory, and speech functions. Instrumentation not only facilitates data collection and storage, but also enables clinicians to draw diagnostic conclusions and make important clinical decisions (Table 4–1).

Because instrumental evaluation has already proven to be a cost-effective and indispensable aid to diagnosis, the need for technology in the voice clinic and laboratory is no longer questioned. Rather, the issues at hand involve determining how to best address three major components of voice pathology diagnosis:

Selecting appropriate instruments and methodologies,

Ensuring proper use of equipment, and

Strengthening data interpretation.

The process through which we derive an *operating clinical hypothesis* remains largely subjective, thus appropriate selection of objective test data is a critical step in confirming or rejecting the hypothesis, and in further developing the clinical profile.

Bless (1993) compiled an extensive list of instrumental measures from which clinicians may select the most appropriate procedures to assess each individual's voice disorder (Table 4–2). This list reflects the current standards of practice in instrumental voice evaluation. Certain measures, such as those providing data on average acoustic and aerodynamic values during speech or other phonatory tasks; physiological ranges of pulmonary function, fundamental frequency, and intensity of voice; or videostroboscopic measures of vocal fold vibratory patterns, typically comprise a core battery for clinical evaluation of all patients within a voice clinic. Standardized protocols should be used in combination with these proce-

TABLE 4–1. Roles of instrumentation in speech analysis.

Functions of Instruments	Uses of Instrumental Data
Inputting physiological phenomena	Making a differential diagnosis
Calculating measurements	Establishing the extent of disease
Transforming signals	Determining the degree of dysphonia
Storing information	Monitoring and documenting changes in structure and function
	Providing prognostic indicators
Interpreting results	Assisting in treatment planning
Displaying data	Enhancing the patient's understanding of the voice problem, and . . .
	Facilitating communication among health care professionals

TABLE 4–2. Instrumental measures of voice.

I. PULMONARY FUNCTION MEASURES
  A. LUNG VOLUMES
      1. Tidal Volume (TV)
      2. Inspiratory Reserve Volume (IRV)
      3. Expiratory Reserve Volume (ERV)
      4. Vital Capacity (VC)
      5. Other Lung Volume/Capacity Measures
  B. FORCED SPIROMETRY
      1. Forced Vital Capacity (FVC)
      2. Flow Volume Loop (FVL)
  C. RESPIRATORY MOVEMENTS
      1. Rib-Cage Excursions
      2. Abdominal Excursions

II. NEUROPHYSIOLOGICAL MEASURES
  A. LARYNGEAL ELECTROMYOGRAPHY (LEMG)
  B. CERVICAL ELECTROMYOGRAPHY (CERVICAL EMG)
  C. PALATAL ELECTROMYOGRAPHY (PALATAL EMG)

III. LARYNGEAL IMAGING MEASURES
  A. STATIC MEASURES
      1. Plain Film Images
      2. Computerized Tomographic Images (CT Scan)
      3. Magnetic Resonance Images (MR Scan)
  B. DYNAMIC MEASURES
      1. Laryngeal Mirror Images
      2. Videoendoscopic Images
      3. Stereofiberscopic Images
      4. Cineradiographic Images
      5. Ultra High Speed Photography Images
      6. Videofluoroscopic Images
      7. Ultrasound Images
      8. Videostroboscopic Images

continued

IV. MEASURES OF VOCAL FOLD CONTACT AREA
    A. ELECTROGLOTTOGRAPHIC SIGNALS (EGG)
    B. PHOTOGLOTTOGRAPHIC SIGNALS (PGG)

V. AERODYNAMIC MEASURES
    A. MEAN AIRFLOW RATE (MFR)
    B. INTRA-ORAL AIR PRESSURE (PO)
    C. GLOTTAL RESISTANCE (PO/MFR)
    D. PHONATORY VOLUME (PV)
    E. PHONATION THRESHOLD PRESSURE (PTP)
    F. NASAL FLOW (VN)
    G. NASAL PRESSURE (PN)
    H. NASAL RESISTANCE (PN/MFRN)

VI. ACOUSTIC MEASURES
    A. MEAN FUNDAMENTAL FREQUENCY (FO)
    B. PHYSIOLOGICAL FREQUENCY RANGE OF PHONATION (PFRP)
    C. STANDARD DEVIATION OF FUNDAMENTAL FREQUENCY (SD FO)
    D. VOCAL INTENSITY (I)
    E. INTENSITY RANGE OF PHONATION (IRP)
    F. FREQUENCY-INTENSITY PROFILE (PHONETOGRAM)
    G. PITCH PERTURBATION (JITTER)
    H. AMPLITUDE PERTURBATION (SHIMMER)
    I. SIGNAL-TO-NOISE RATIO (SNR)
    J. NASALANCE
    K. VOICE ONSET TIME (VOT)
    L. SOUND SPECTROGRAPHIC ANALYSIS (SSA)
    M. LONG-TIME AVERAGE SPECTRA (LTAS)
    N. DURATIONAL MEASURES

VII. MEASURES OF VISUAL AND/OR AUDITORY PERFORMANCE
    A. AUDIO RECORDINGS
    B. FULL-FACE OR FULL-BODY VIDEO RECORDINGS

Source: Adapted from "Vocal Function Assessment" by D. Bless, 1993. Presentation at Phonosurgery Symposium, Madison, WI, with permission.

dures to permit valid and reliable pre- and post-treatment comparisons, and comparisons with normative data. Although there is no consensus about which protocols most effectively elicit the necessary diagnostic information, it is generally recognized that individual institutions and centers must be consistent in their use of equipment, procedures, and protocols. Several sample protocols have been included in the appendixes.

Minor modifications of these protocols might be necessary as dictated by patient's age, cognitive abilities, sensory limitations, physical condition, or psychological state. Most patients, however, are able to perform these tasks without difficulty, especially if the clinician adapts elicitation techniques and/or reinforcement systems as required.

SELECTING THE APPROPRIATE TOOLS

New technologies in diagnostic imaging and clinical evaluation have enabled practitioners to more accurately relate structure and function to the sound of the voice. Appropriate equipment selection is essential to ensure valid measures of vocal function.

Magnetic Resonance Imaging (MRI)

Unlike plain-film radiologic techniques, MRI uses a magnetic field that causes protons in the body to align themselves and spin parallel to the direction of a magnet (Figure 4–1). When radio frequencies are applied to the magnetic field, the protons react by absorbing and emitting energy (resonance) as they relocate and then return to their aligned positions. On the basis of measurements about the disturbed protons (proton density and proton relaxation times, Tl and T2), an image is generated that provides information regarding the physical properties of the tissues in which the protons lie.

The procedure, conducted by a technician and interpreted by a radiologist, can be performed in hospitals, clinics, outpatient imaging centers, or even mobile scanning units. A recent trend toward shared mobile scanners has enabled smaller communities to avail themselves of this and other sophisticated technologies, while sharing the costs of equipment.

Total scanning time for an MRI ranges from 30 to 90 minutes, depending on the type of examination to be performed (e.g., head scan, neck scan, head and neck scan). Although the procedure is painless and noninvasive, people with claustrophobia might encounter difficulty if special precautions are not taken (Figure 4–2). In these cases, sedation, the use of special eyeglasses (prism lenses that direct the patient's vision outside of the MRI encasement), and/or covering the eyes with a cloth are effective strategies that can relieve anxiety.

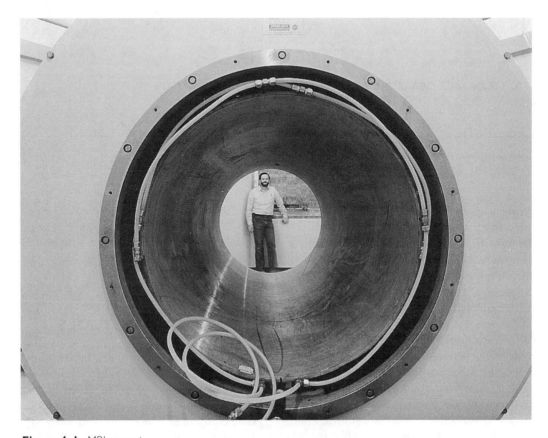

Figure 4–1. MRI magnet.

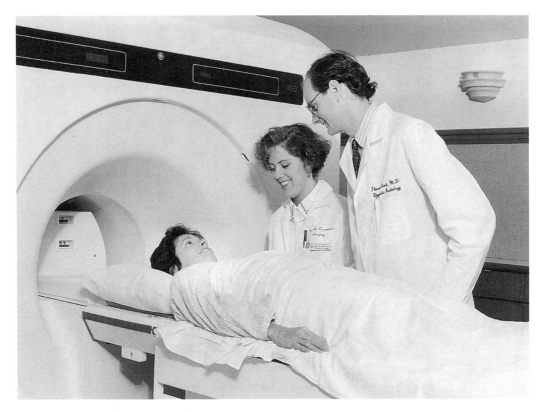

Figure 4–2. MRI procedure: patient about to undergo scan.

There are no known health risks associated with MRI, although the long-term side effects remain unknown. The technique is usually contraindicated in patients with ferrous materials inside the body such as pacemakers, neurostimulators, metal plates, cochlear implants, brain or blood vessel clips, or metal fragments in the head, eye, or skin. Overall, the dollar costs of MRI scanning are quite high relative to the expenses incurred from other types of diagnostic imaging procedures.

Through MR scanning it has become possible to visualize the soft tissue structures of the head and neck in exquisite detail (Figure 4–3). Two- and three-dimensional images of the head and neck regions are used to detect and diagnose a variety of abnormalities that can impair the human voice. Such abnormalities may be related to a central nervous system disorder (e.g., Parkinson's disease), a muscular disease (e.g., myasthenia gravis), or a laryngeal tumor.

Computerized Tomography (CT)

The CT scan can provide incomparable diagnostic information to the laryngologist in preoperative assessments of head and neck tumors. For example, during a preoperative evaluation of a patient with a laryngeal malignancy, the surgeon seeks information to determine the size and extent of a tumor and any possible invasion into cartilaginous structures. In such a case, the CT scan is comparable to MRI in its capability to demonstrate extension of tumors into the soft tissues of the neck, lymph node metastasis and invasion into ossified cartilage (Castelijns et al., 1988; Weissman & Curtin, 1995).

Following surgery or radiation therapy, the CT scan is generally the preferred modality for monitoring the effects of treatments because of its capability to differentiate tumor from surrounding edema (Walker-

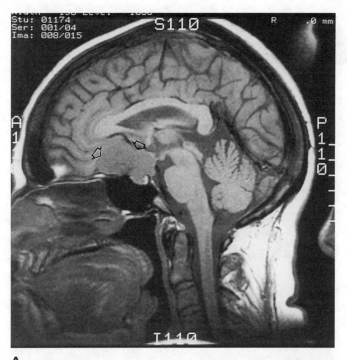

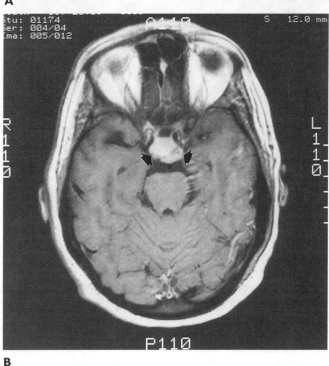

Figure 4–3. Magnetic Resonance Images (MRI) showing details of tumor. **A.** Sagittal T1-weighted (precontrast) MRI showing lobulated mass arising from skull base. Tumor is isodense with brain tissue. **B.** Axial T1-weighted (postcontrast) MRI showing homogeneous enhancement of skull-base tumor.

Patient 4–1: MRI / Brainstem
Congenital Abnormality

This patient was a 63-year-old female who had experienced progressive difficulty with dysarthria and swallowing for over 2 years. Because her speech had become unintelligible, she communicated through writing.

Initial evaluation revealed numerous characteristics of flaccid dysarthria involving the VII, X, and XII cranial nerves. Specifically, she demonstrated an asymmetrical smile at rest, difficulty rounding the lips, an absent gag reflex, hypernasality, nasal emissions, weak cough, weak glottic closure, a prolonged open phase in the vocal fold vibratory cycle, atrophy and fasciculations of the tongue, and weak tongue movements on lateralization and protrusion.

Following speech, laryngologic, and neurological evaluations, the patient was referred for an MRI scan. The findings revealed an unusual appearance of the craniocervical junction, in which the cervical spinal cord and medulla were crowded (Figure 4–4). The diagnosis was Arnold-Chiari 1 deformity. Subsequent to surgical intervention, the patient regained functional communication and swallowing abilities.

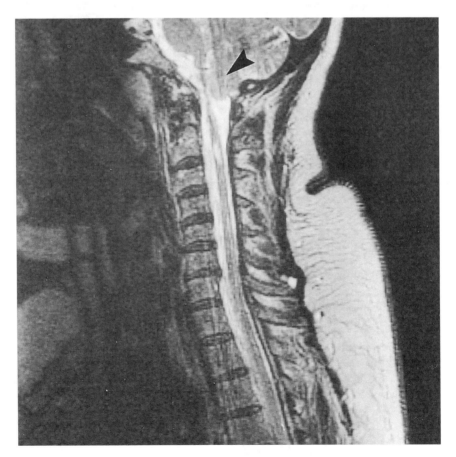

Figure 4–4. MRI image: Arnold Chiari I malformation. Sagittal T2-weighted image of the cervical spine shows extension of the cerebellar tonsil inferiorly through the foramen magnum, with crowding of the medulla.

Batson & Purdy, 1991). Similarly, in cases of acute laryngeal trauma, CT scanning has proven extremely effective in identifying occult fractures of the thyroid cartilage or cricoid ring and dislocations of the arytenoid. Symptoms warranting CT scanning after acute trauma might include laryngeal tenderness, endolaryngeal edema, and small to medium hematomas (Schaefer, 1991).

A CT scan is actually an x-ray that provides a cross-sectional image of the body. The CT scanner, which uses an x-ray tube that moves in a circle around the patient, interfaces with a computer and generates a visual image. The CT procedure is performed by an x-ray technician and the results are read and interpreted by a radiologist. The time required to perform a CT scan is generally less than for an MRI, usually ranging from 20 to 40 minutes.

There may be slightly greater health risks associated with CT relative to MRI because it is a radiological study. Of course, the procedure should be avoided by pregnant women. The procedure might be contraindicated in some people who have allergies to iodine as an intravenous contrast dye is sometimes used to enhance imaging and to maximize technical quality.

When the diagnostic information offered by CT and MRI is considered comparable, CT scanning is usually chosen, for the dollar costs of CT are approximately half those for MRI. In difficult cases, however, both CT and MRI might be required to correlate and confirm test findings. The overall effectiveness of this diagnostic imaging technique, combined with its relatively lower cost, have made CT a widely used imaging modality available in most hospital sites today.

Videofluoroscopy

Problems relating to gastroesophageal reflux or esophageal dysmotility can be detected with videofluoroscopic examination. The testing procedure involves drinking barium materials that have a specific texture and consistency (thin liquid, thick liquid, puree or paste, or solids). The barium used to outline the soft tissues in the swallowing tract enhances visualization of the swallowing structures.

As a patient swallows, an x-ray demonstrating the dynamics of swallowing function appears on a video screen. During a modified barium swallow (Figure 4–6), the bolus is observed as it travels through the

---

Patient 4–2: CT Scan / Supraglottic Cancer

A 57-year-old male factory worker reported a 3-month history of sore throat and hoarseness. He had a 100-pack-per-year history of tobacco use.

Indirect examination of the larynx revealed an invasive, exophytic mass involving the left pyriform fossa. In addition to endoscopy and biopsy, a CT neck scan was performed to assist in tumor staging and to determine if there was invasion of cartilage or evidence of cervical adenopathy.

Axial images were obtained from the level of the clavicular heads to the nasopharynx. Radiographically, the examination demonstrated a mass in the left pyriform fossa (Figure 4–5). There was no evidence of cartilaginous or bony invasion; however, adenopathy was identified in the left neck.

The tumor was diagnosed as a $T_3N_1M_0$ (Stage III) squamous cell carcinoma of the supraglottic larynx. This patient had preoperative radiation therapy and subsequently underwent a total laryngectomy and left radical neck dissection.

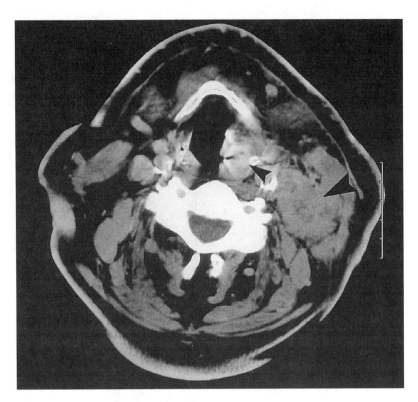

Figure 4–5. CT image: Axial CT image through the larynx, showing a 2 cm mass in the left pyriform fossa (*small arrow*) and a large nodal mass deep in the sternocleidomastoid muscle (*large arrow*). The findings are consistent with metastatic carcinoma of the larynx.

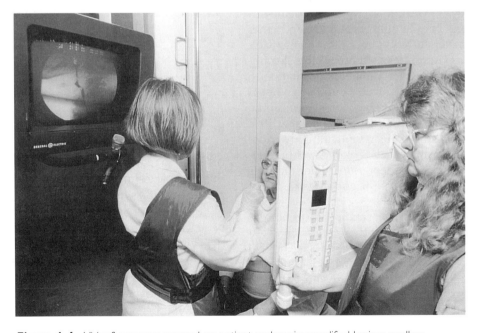

Figure 4–6. Videofluoroscopy procedure: patient undergoing modified barium swallow.

upper passageway—the oral cavity, the oropharynx, and the hypopharynx, to the level of the upper esophageal sphincter. Should aspiration occur, a straying bolus can be seen entering the larynx and airway. Other problems such as pooling in the pyriform sinuses or timing difficulties might also be demonstrated during testing. More refined measures can be made by digitizing video images of the examination and defining times and locations of the swallowing events with the aid of a computer program.

Additional information can be obtained when an esophagram is performed in combination with a modified barium swallow. The esophagram is a radiographic image of the esophagus, from the upper to lower esophageal sphincter, that can identify structural deviations or motility problems in the lower swallowing tract. Procedurally, the esophagram involves consuming a greater amount of barium to more fully distend the esophageal walls, and, as above, making a radiographic image of the esophagus (Figure 4–7).

For the laryngeal speaker, the use of motion fluoroscopy can aid in the assessment of adductory and abductory glottic patterns, changes in vertical larynx height, plane differences between the vocal folds, and other parameters of vocal tract movements (Colton & Casper, 1990). Although this last application can offer valuable information to the evaluation process, subtle laryngeal problems such as plane differences can be difficult to distinguish, particularly in a nonaspirating patient. Only a highly experienced examiner who has reviewed literally hundreds of videofluoroscopic studies is likely to be capable of judging these obscured dimensions.

Videofluoroscopic testing is generally performed by at least two professionals—a speech pathologist who conducts the test and an x-ray technician who operates the radiographic equipment. In some medical centers, a radiologist might also be involved in the study. Testing generally lasts from 15 to 30 minutes.

Although patients generally dislike the taste of barium, there is no pain or discom-

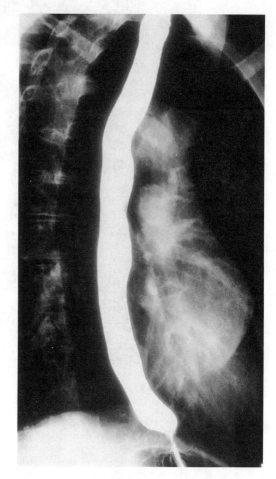

Figure 4–7. Esophagram image.

fort associated with the examinations. Since fluoroscopy does involve use of radiation, testing is contraindicated in pregnant women and patients subject to the health risks common to radiographic procedures. Videofluoroscopic testing is available in many, but not all, hospital sites.

Videofluoroscopic testing has proven beneficial to many patients with voice disorders who report symptoms of dysphagia or gastroesophageal reflux disease (GERD). Individuals with voice problems who are at risk for swallowing problems are those with neurological conditions, head and neck tumors, gastroesophageal reflux, thyroid problems, diabetes mellitus, and the geriatric population.

Although used predominantly in the assessment of swallowing disorders, videofluoroscopic technology can also be applied to the assessment of certain speech and voice disorders. For instance, in patients with velopharyngeal dysfunction, radiographic studies can assist in assessing both the degree and pattern of velopharyngeal closure (McWilliams, Morris, & Shelton, 1990). In an alaryngeal speaker, dimensions such as upper esophageal sphincter hyperconstriction and air pocketing can be evaluated using this technique (Salmon & Mount, 1991).

Videostroboscopy

Whereas classical laryngeal endoscopy allows practitioners to inspect the vocal folds and related structures visually, laryngeal videostroboscopy provides additional information regarding vocal fold vibration. Consequently, the technique of videostroboscopy combines a thorough examination of the laryngeal structures for asymmetries, tumors, mass lesions, webbing, granulomatous disease, or other pathologies, and of the vibratory patterns produced during phonation.

The principles of videostroboscopy have been discussed by Hirano and Bless (1993). During videostroboscopy, different points in the vocal fold vibratory cycle are sampled (i.e., illuminated by light flashes emitted by the stroboscope) across successive vocal fold vibratory cycles. The stroboscope emits pulses of light at rates that are 2–3 Hz

---

Patient 4–3: Videofluoroscopy/ Gastroesophageal Reflux

This female patient, a 55-year-old bartender, was seen initially in the Voice Clinic for evaluation of hoarseness and swallowing problems. She complained of intermittent raspiness, vocal fatigue, a globus sensation ("feeling a lump in the throat"), and the inability to clear foods from the hypopharyngeal area during swallowing. She had a medical history of insulin-dependent diabetes, which had been diagnosed 7 years before.

On physical examination, the patient presented with erythema in the posterior larynx.

Videostroboscopic evaluation revealed complete glottic closure, a significant degree of supraglottic constriction associated with phonation, and interarytenoid mucus stranding.

Videofluoroscopic evaluation demonstrated normal oral and pharyngeal motility with intake of liquids and semi-solids. No aspiration was noted and there were no structural abnormalities within the oropharyngeal tract. However, the esophagram did indicate a severe esophageal dysmotility with extremely diminished primary and secondary wave and a significant amount of tertiary contractions. Gastroesophageal reflux was also documented during the evaluation.

On the basis of the patient's history, the physical findings, and the results of the esophagram, it was suspected that reflux of gastric contents into the pharynx was the primary cause of the patient's hoarseness secondary to mucosal irritation from the GERD. Periods of vocal abuse at work, and muscle misuse secondary to the GERD, were also suggested by her history. She was initially asked to implement antireflux measures and observe vocal hygiene suggestions, then return for follow-up. The information gained regarding the esophageal dysmotility problems was shared with her physician in the Diabetes Clinic to determine if anything might be done to alleviate those problems.

different from the patient's phonatory fundamental frequency. Stroboscopy produces an optical illusion when the human eye fuses the fragmented laryngeal images into a perceptually complete vibratory movement. The appearance is of slow-motion vibration (Figure 4–8A). Since the images are only appearances, the vibratory patterns must be inferred by a knowledgeable specialist. Most stroboscopes also allow the examiner to control the stroboscopic light pulses so they illuminate the same portion of each vibratory cycle (phase-locked setting). This setting provides an impression of regularity or periodicity from one cycle to the next, by the degree to which the image remains still, or, in the case of an aperiodic vibratory pattern, by the degree of perceived visual "jitter" (Figure 4–8B).

Aberrant vibratory patterns revealed by stroboscopy may indicate vocal fold stiffness or adynamic segments, mucosal edema, decreased muscle tone or flaccidity, or other vibratory impairments. Previously undetected laryngeal pathologies (e.g., sulcus vocalis, pseudocysts, prenodular vocal fold mucosal swelling) can frequently be identified and diagnosed through the com-

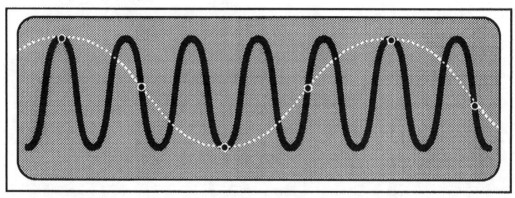

A

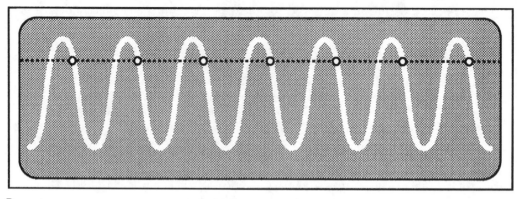

B

Figure 4–8. Principles of stroboscopy: **A.** If the strobe light is set to flash slightly off the f_0, a slow-motion image will be perceived. **B.** If the strobe light is set to flash at the same frequency as the phonatory f_0, the image will give the impression of a still-frame. (Reprinted with permission from M. D. Morrison & L. A. Rammage et al., 1994, p. 35. *The management of voice disorders*. London: Chapman & Hall Medical/San Diego: Singular Publishing Group, Inc.)

bined use of magnification and stroboscopy. The specific parameters assessed are reflected in the video-stroboscopic score form (Appendix 4–1).

The procedure can be adapted to either a standard transoral rigid telescopic endoscope or a flexible fiberoptic naso-pharyngo-laryngoscope. Different lenses vary in their degree of magnification, clarity of image, and visual perspective. Rigid endoscopes generally provide the greatest magnification, illumination and image detail (Figure 4–9). During rigid endoscopy, the patient is asked to phonate the vowel /i/ and then vary pitch, loudness, and the rate of production (diadochokinesis-DDK). Naso-endoscopy utilizes fiberoptic technology and has the advantage of providing a panoramic view of the larynx and sampling

ongoing speech as well as vowel productions (Figure 4–10). The flexible scope can also be used to observe velopharyngeal closure patterns as part of the examination protocol. Care should be taken when comparisons are made between images obtained with different laryngoscopes; in particular, the examiner-judge needs to be aware of different perspectives and perceptions of the laryngeal image offered by the rigid and flexible scopes (Sodersten & Lindestad, 1992).

The total duration of an examination usually ranges from 10 to 20 minutes depending on the procedure, the skill of the examiner, and the cooperation of the patient. The testing is generally performed by a speech pathologist, although some laryngologists perform the examinations routinely. Other

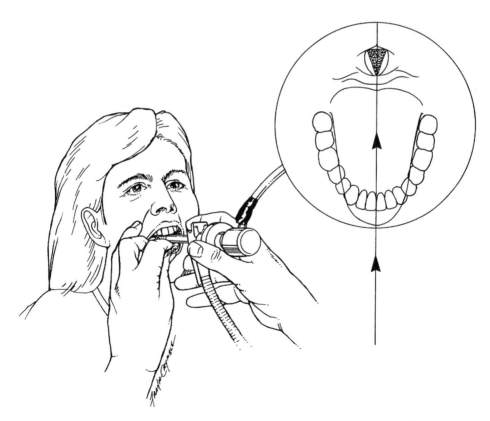

Figure 4–9. Transoral examination for video-laryngostroboscopy, using a rigid endoscope. (Reprinted with permission from M. D. Morrison & L. A. Rammage et al., 1994, p. 33. *The management of voice disorders.* London: Chapman & Hall Medical/San Diego: Singular Publishing Group, Inc.)

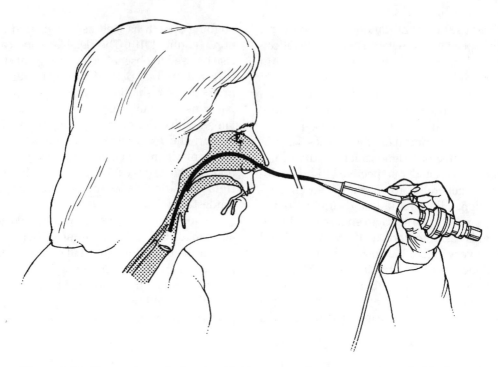

Figure 4–10. Transnasal examination for video-laryngoscopy/stroboscopy, using a flexible fiberoptic scope. (Reprinted with permission from M. D. Morrison & L. A. Rammage et al., 1994, p. 31. *The management of voice disorders.* London: Chapman & Hall Medical/San Diego: Singular Publishing Group, Inc.)

voice care team members (e.g., a singing specialist) might be present during the examination. However, it is not necessary to view the videostroboscopic sample at the time of testing, for the images are permanently recorded on videotape. In fact, ideally, formal scoring of the videostroboscopic images is conducted post-hoc, by judge-clinicians who are "blinded" to the potentially biasing factors provided by patient history, test results, and sound of the voice (Teitler, 1992). Further, accurate and reliable interpretation of the stroboscopic images depends on use of a consistent protocol that includes examination of vibratory patterns during a variety of phonatory tasks, representing a variety of timing-duration, intensity, and fundamental frequency conditions (Hirano & Bless, 1993). A sample protocol for video-laryngostrobscopic evaluation is provided in Appendix 4–2.

Videostroboscopy is available in many specialty voice clinics located in hospitals and clinic settings. The growing popularity of this technique has significantly increased its application in private practices and has made this procedure an essential component of the vocal function laboratory.

The endoscopic procedures used during videostroboscopy are relatively noninvasive and minimally uncomfortable for the patient. Since some people with a hyperactive gag reflex might require the use of a topical anesthetic during rigid endoscopy, it is important to question the patient regarding possible allergic reactions. Xylocaine, a topical anesthetic sometimes used to numb the posterior tongue and oropharynx prior to laryngeal examination, can facilitate visualization of the larynx. The use of a topical anesthetic would be contraindicated, however, in a patient who has experienced a previous allergic reaction to lidocaine (e.g., during dental work). These instances are extremely rare and do not usually prevent visualization of the larynx in the hands of an experienced examiner.

Patient 4–4: Videostroboscopy/Professional Voice User

This 47-year-old, 4 ft. 11 in. 185-lb minister complained of having lost her ability to sing. She was particularly concerned about her loss of vocal range and inability to sustain notes, for these difficulties had limited her participation in community performances.

Onset of her vocal difficulties had begun in January following an upper respiratory infection. She reported coughing and clearing her throat excessively at that time; she still felt the need to do so in November when she came into the clinic for evaluation. She reported that, typically, her singing voice was worse early in the morning, improved somewhat during the course of the day, and worsened again by evening.

Following a case history interview, the patient was administered a battery of vocal function tests that included aerodynamic, acoustic, and videostroboscopic assessments. Only the findings from the videostroboscopic study are reported below.

Videostroboscopic evaluation using a rigid endoscope and made during phonation of the sustained vowel /i/ revealed symmetrical laryngeal structures and regular vocal fold movements at varying pitch and loudness levels. Amplitude was judged to be normal bilaterally, as was mucosal wave. Nevertheless, several abnormalities were noted. The first problem was evident in the anterior portion of the membranous area of the vocal folds. Bilateral edema was noted during vocal fold approximation, particularly at high pitch levels. During high-pitched phonation, the edematous segment was the only area that closed, leaving a clear nodal diathesis during the closed phase of the glottal cycle. An irregular margin, not unlike a small contact granuloma, was visualized immediately posterior to the left vocal process of the arytenoid (Figure 4–11).

On the basis of these findings, in combination with the patient's history and other medical and physiological test results, it appeared that her problems were due at least in part to poor vocal hygiene and gastroesophageal reflux. A vocal hygiene program and an antireflux protocol were established for the patient and she was asked to return for reevaluation in 1 month.

Videoendoscopy

Only recently has the value of diagnostic testing by videoendoscopy been fully recognized in voice care clinics. Many voice care teams, however, routinely make use of this method to assess the potential benefits of various phonosurgical and behavioral management techniques.

The method involves the use of either a rigid transoral endoscope or a flexible transnasal endoscope connected to a video system to allow imaging of the larynx. Both laryngeal manual compression tests and diagnostic probe therapy techniques can be used to elicit voice improvements.

Most commonly, the speech pathologist conducts this type of stimulability testing at the end of the videostroboscopic evaluation. Both the speech pathologist and laryngologist can assess the auditory perceptual and physiological changes that occur.

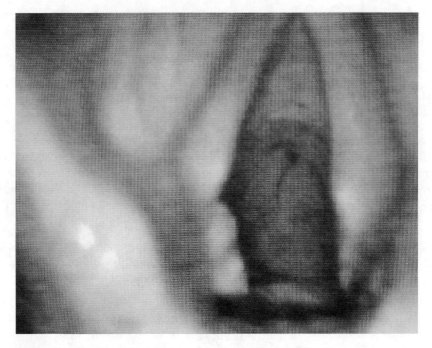

Figure 4–11. Video-print from laryngostroboscopic image, showing contact granuloma on left vocal fold in the typical interarytenoid position.

VOCAL FUNCTION TESTING

During vocal function testing, the voice care team administers a comprehensive battery of tests designed to evaluate phonatory function. Within this diagnostic battery are both instrumental and noninstrumental examinations of voice, including measurements of phonatory ability and laryngeal movement, and perceptual, aerodynamic, and acoustic evaluations or electromyography. Among the authors who have described these examinations in detail are Hirano (1981), Bless (1991a, 1991b), and Baken (1987). With the exception of laryngeal electromyography (EMG), these diagnostic procedures are routinely performed by the speech pathologist in the vocal function laboratory.

Classic tools of the clinical examination such as the electroglottograph, Respitrace, spectrograph, and physiological data acquisition and analysis systems provide objective, specific information regarding vocal function. Together with scaling techniques,

these instrumental analyses allow clinicians to delineate respiratory and laryngeal functions, examine phonatory patterns, and help determine the etiology of the dysphonia. Furthermore, they provide objective documentation supporting the efficacy of surgical, pharmacological, behavioral, or radiation therapy treatments.

Acoustic Measures

The voice clinician now has access to a large selection of computer-based programs dedicated to measurement of the acoustic signal of speech. Most software programs designed for clinical use are capable of providing on-line (immediate feedback) displays and values for a variety of acoustic features: averaged fundamental frequency (f_0); intensity (I); intonation patterns and values; and speech sound durations. More sophisticated systems that may be adapted for clinical use provide additional features such as measures of vocal harmonics, formant frequencies, voice onset times (VOT), and selected measures of perturbation in frequency (jitter) and/or intensity (shimmer), and signal-to-noise ratios (SNR). Examples of user-friendly systems for clinical application include Visi-Pitch® (Kay Elemetrics), Speech Viewer (IBM Corp.), and Voice Identification PM Pitch Analyzer. More sophisticated programs, used for basic and clinical research, allow the clinician to examine and analyze the speech signal in greater detail by using specialized acoustic filters, algorithms, synthesis, and spectral analysis techniques. CSpeech (Milenkovic, University of Wisconsin); CSRE (Avaaz Innovations, Inc.); and CSL (Kay Elemetrics) are just three examples of sophisticated acoustic analysis software that may be used for detailed analysis of clinical data.

Objective instrumental measures of the acoustic speech signal allow the clinician to quantify important aspects of physiological function and may be used to corroborate or supplement subjective and perceptual measures. As with other clinical regimens, the exact protocol used to evaluate the acoustic speech signal varies from clinic to clinic. A sample protocol for acoustic and prosodic assessment is provided in Appendix 4–3.

Most clinicians would agree that acoustic measures of f_0 and intensity should be included as part of the standard descriptive profile of a patient's voice. Averaged values of f_0 and intensity of speech contribute important information regarding a patient's typical or habitual voice use profile, whereas maximum performance ranges of these acoustic features (physiological ranges) provide important data on the anatomical integrity and/or physiological capability of the laryngeal structure. Normative data exist for comparison with clinical values (Baken, 1987; Bless, Biever, Campos, Glaze, & Peppard, 1989; Hirano, 1981). Changes in F_0 and intensity that contribute suprasegmental features of intonation and stress can be measured acoustically to document and provide feedback regarding speech patterns that may contribute to perceptual impressions of flat, monotone speech (giving the impression of boredom/fatigue) or exaggerated/irratic pro-

sodic styles (giving the impression of bizarreness). Observations of the signal during gradual f_0 or intensity changes can also help describe voice problems, especially in cases of subtle neurological signs or technical misuse (e.g., in singers). Comparison of habitual levels of f_0 or intensity, with values obtained during spontaneous or vegetative vocalizations (e.g., laughing, coughing) or measures made under special probe conditions (e.g., masking, sodium amytal, hypnosis, emotive expression) can provide invaluable diagnostic and treatment information. A phonetogram plots physiological ranges of f_0 and intensity against each other so their profiles and interactive functions can be documented (Figure 4–12). The complex relationships among intensity, f_0, and subglottal pressure are recognized as critical components in defining vocal function (Holmberg, Hillman, & Perkell, 1988; Titze, 1991a)

Acoustic analysis programs can facilitate accurate measurement of rate, duration, and fluency-continuity aspects of speech and phonation. These speech production features provide further valuable diagnostic information regarding the integrity, function, and use of the speech and vocal apparatus. Measurement of maximum phonation time (MPT) on a standard vowel provides information regarding the integrity of the glottic valving system and/or respiratory support, and several sources of normative data for this measure exist (Bless et al., 1989; Hirano, 1981; Kent, Kent, & Rosenbek, 1987). Spectrographic displays can provide the detail necessary for accurate measures of laryngeal diadochokinetics, speaking rate, phrase length, unusual prosody features (e.g., vocal tremor), and breaks in fluency or continuity, for example, the number and duration of phonation breaks associated with spasmodic dysphonia.

Finally, acoustic analysis systems have been used in some clinics to provide objective measures of the acoustic spectrum that contributes to voice quality. Although numerous caveats must be observed when acoustic spectra are interpreted for clinical implications, this tool has been used suc-

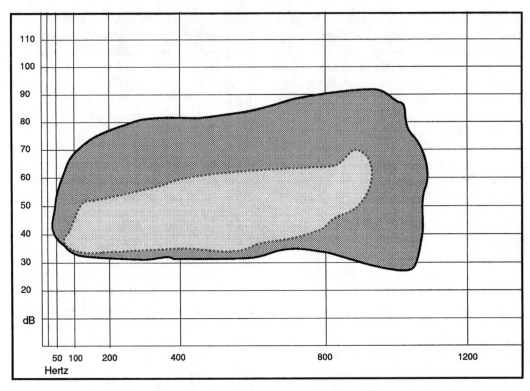

Figure 4–12. Phonetogram plots intensity (I) (*vertical axis*) against f_0 (*horizontal axis*) and demonstrates changes in interactive ranges for I and f_0 pretreatment (*light shading*) and posttreatment (*dark shading*). (Reprinted with permission from M. D. Morrison & L. A. Rammage et al., 1994, p. 12. *The management of voice disorders.* London: Chapman & Hall Medical/San Diego: Singular Publishing Group, Inc.)

cessfully to document acoustic features such as dominance of f_0 and excessive noise—especially in the upper frequency region (often associated with "breathy" or "whispery" quality and inadequate glottic closure) (Figure 4–13A); or high intensity regions in the harmonic or formant structure, such as the strived-for "singer's formant" (Figure 4–13B) (Rammage, 1992; Sundberg, 1987). Most programs provide "summary" values of perturbation, signal-to-noise ratio (or harmonics-to-noise ratio) that can be used to demonstrate treatment changes, as long as production features such as intensity and f_0 are controlled carefully.

Aerodynamic Measures

Aerodynamic measures of voice, like acoustic measures, provide clinically relevent information about laryngeal function that can be obtained with a noninvasive approach. Clinical measures of phonatory and/or nasal flow rates and flow volumes are most commonly obtained with a face mask attached to a flow transducing unit (Figure 4–14). A pneumotachograph, hot-wire anemometer, plethysmograph, or electro-aerometer may be used to transduce the aerodynamic signal to an electrical one that can be further analyzed and converted to standard units (cc per second; ml per second) and compared with norms. Mean phonatory flow rate (MFR) measured during production of a steady-state open vowel provides an estimate of glottic impedance, since oral resistance is at a minimum when the upper vocal tract is open: as such the primary factors affecting flow rates are respiratory effort and glottic impedance. High phonatory flow rates are generally indicative of poor glottic valving, whereas low phonatory flow rates

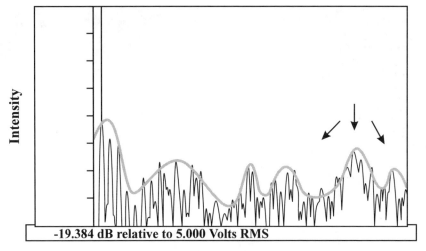

A

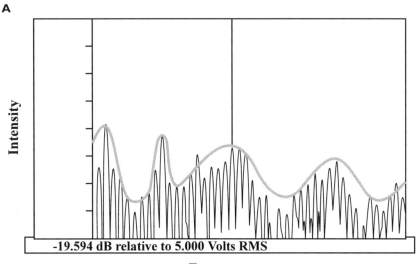

B

Figure 4–13. Schematized acoustic spectra, adapted from CSpeech analyses. Acoustic spectra demonstrate intensities and frequencies/bandwidths of vocal harmonics and/or formants. **A.** In "breathy" voices, typical acoustic spectra may demonstrate the dominance of f_0 (cursor: first peak on left), poorly defined formants, and wide bands of noise especially in the upper frequencies (*arrows*). **B.** Relatively intense harmonics in the mid and upper frequency ranges are typical of periodic, clear voices. Intense harmonics in high frequencies is related closely to rapid closure of the vocal folds during the vibratory cycles. A "singer's formant" may be formed by vocal tract adjustments that enhance the third and fourth formants (*cursor*).

indicate hypervalving, but may also reflect low intensity and/or poor respiratory support. Phonatory flow volume may also be measured to provide a value for cumulative flow (cc or ml) during a maximum performance test such as MPT, or to compare with measures of respiratory function such as forced vital capacity.

Pressure is a measure of force and can be used to derive indicators of phonatory effort. In the clinic, glottic pressure values can be inferred from intra-oral pressures ob-

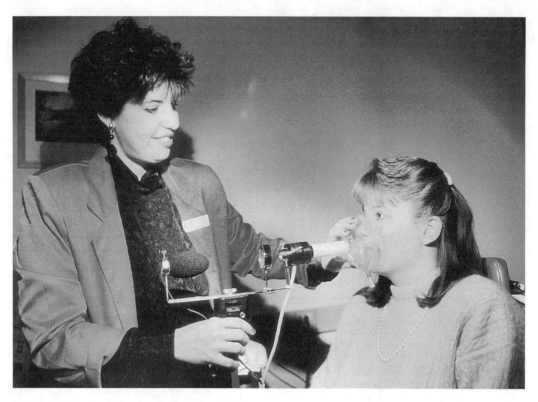

Figure 4–14. Aerodynamic testing using partial face mask, attached to flow and pressure transducers.

tained with a small plastic tube, placed intra-orally, and attached to a pressure transducer. As described by Smitheran and Hixon (1981), the subglottic pressures can be inferred from intra-oral pressures (P_0) generated during the lip closure for /p/; and the glottal flow rates ($\mathring{V}$) can be estimated from adjacent vowels. Thus, during carefully elicited productions of /pæpæpæpæ . . . /, one estimates averaged subglottal pressures and phonatory flow rates, and laryngeal resistance can be derived by: $P_0/(\mathring{V})$, to indicate laryngeal "effort." Phonation threshold pressures (PTP) are readily obtained during aerodynamic testing, and can provide clinically relevant data defining the minimum force required to initiate phonation, under varying production and vocal health conditions (Titze, 1991a; Verdolini, Titze, & Druker, 1990).

Because flow rates and pressures are influenced by phonation frequency and intensity (and/or effort), care must be taken

to elicit productions that are controlled for these production factors.

A sample protocol for aerodynamic assessment of vocal function is provided in Appendix 4–4.

Other Measures of Vocal Function

Measures of Cycle-by-Cycle Phonatory Patterns

When an inverse-filtering process is applied to phonatory flow measures to effectively eliminate effects of the vocal tract filter on the volume-velocity flow waveform, then **flow glottograms** are derived. The Rothenberg face mask (Rothenberg, 1973) performs this function. The resultant waveform primarily reflects fine details regarding the effects of vocal fold movements on the flow waveform on a cycle-by-cycle basis, and can be used to infer important information regarding the biomechanics of phonation (Hertegard, Gauffin, & Karlsson, 1992; Rothenberg, 1973, 1977, 1981).

The **electroglottograph** (EGG) can also provide information about vocal fold vibratory patterns, by measuring the impedance at the glottis as a low-voltage current is passed between two electrodes. These electrodes are held firmly on the surface of the neck over the thyroid lamina bilaterally. When the vocal folds are in maximal contact, impedance is maximally low, whereas an open glottis offers high impedance. EGG is used to estimate vocal fold contact area and f_0, and some attempts have been made to interpret the resultant waveforms in greater detail to predict pathology and to compare with other clinical measures such as flow glottograms (Baer, Titze, & Yoshioka, 1983; Baken, 1987; Childers et al., 1983; Dromey, Stathopoulos, & Sapienza, 1992; Lee & Childers, 1991; Titze, 1990). However, there is still no consensus regarding the exact interpretation of EGG waveform shapes or their clincial diagnostic value. Some difficulties have been reported in obtaining reliable data from certain patients, in particular, women and children, individuals with enough adipose tissue in the neck to distort the signal, or patients with mucus strands that mimic vocal fold contact areas during open portions of the vibratory cycle.

In contrast to EGG, which indicates degree of vocal fold contact, **photoglottography** (PGG) measures the amount of light transmitted through the glottis during open phases of the vibratory cycle and thus provides information about phonatory patterns from a different perspective. The hardware and signals associated with EGG and PGG are demonstrated in Figure 4–15. Since PGG requires more sophisticated hardware and data processing, and is considerably more invasive than EGG, it is used less commonly in clinical settings.

Measures of Respiratory and Speech-Breathing Patterns

Since the respiratory system provides the raw power source for speech in the form of airflow, the final (radiated) speech signal must be interpreted as a product of passive and active respiratory forces combined with relevant valving and vocal tract shaping functions that occur in the larynx, pharynx, and mouth during speech, as well as biomechanical and aerodynamic interactions between the various systems. Basic measures of respiratory function can be used to indicate the degree to which the respiratory system contributes to a voice disorder.

Respiratory measures of forced vital capacity and tidal flow and volume can be made using a variety of instruments typically available in pulmonary function labs, but in the voice clinic, the flow transducer and other hardware used for phonatory flow measures can be readily adapted for this purpose. Forced vital capacity measures, made during maximum exhalation following maximum inhalation, provide the clinician with a value that can be compared against well-documented normative data. The patient with a greatly reduced vital capacity may demonstrate short maximum phonation times, short speech phrases, and a weak or aesthenic voice with reduced intensity due to difficulty achieving adequate subglottal pressure during speech. The normal aging process, along with a variety of diseases affecting pulmonary tissue and function may contribute to low vital capacity. A computer-generated flow-versus-volume loop provides further information regarding ventilatory impairment due to a variety of pulmonary diseases (Slavit, 1995).

Measures of tidal flow and volume may be compared with speech-breathing patterns, to differentiate between voice problems due primarily to respiratory functions and those reflecting primary laryngeal problems or more generalized speech and voice dysfunction.

Speech breathing functions can be investigated further in terms of respiratory movement patterns (kinematics) of the rib cage and abdomen. Based on detailed investigations by Hixon and his colleagues (Hixon, 1987) on the most accurate means for mea-

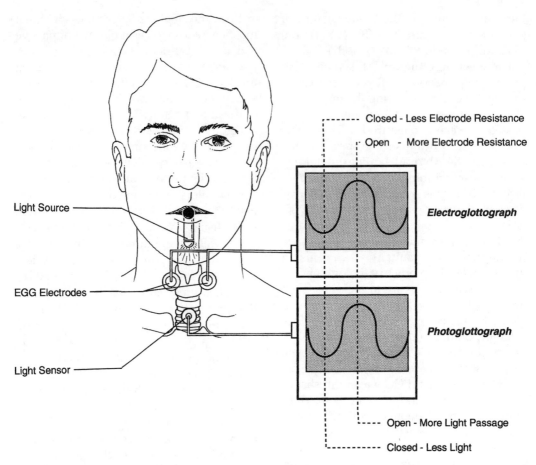

Light Source

EGG Electrodes

Light Sensor

Closed - Less Electrode Resistance

Open - More Electrode Resistance

Electroglottograph

Photoglottograph

Open - More Light Passage

Closed - Less Light

Figure 4–15. Hardware and idealized waveforms for electroglottography (EGG) and photoglottography (PGG). (Reprinted with permission from M. D. Morrison & L. A. Rammage et al., 1994, p. 44. *The management of voice disorders.* London: Chapman & Hall Medical/San Diego: Singular Publishing Group, Inc.)

suring speech breathing patterns, motion-motion graphs of the relative movements of two portions of the chest wall (rib cage versus abdomen) can be made using magnetometry or dedicated instruments, such as Respitrace (inductive plethysmography) (Figure 4–16). Since the complementary measures of respiratory pressure (force) provided by the two primary speech-breathing areas can only be made with invasive procedures, the relative contributions of the rib cage and abdomen to support speech breathing are usually inferred from kinematic measures in the clinical setting.

Although there are no contraindications for vocal function testing, it does require the patient's cooperation. Physical factors

(e.g., fatigue, facial deformities), emotional problems, or cognitive limitations can occasionally prevent the clinician from obtaining accurate or complete data, particularly on maximum performance tasks. This is uncommon, however, and even children as young as 4 years old can perform the necessary vocal tasks when provided with appropriate instructions, modeling, and reinforcement.

Total examination time and dollar costs for an analysis of vocal function vary among sites, depending on the purpose of the examination (test protocol) and the type and availability of laboratory equipment. In general, the procedures are noninvasive and permit data collection without any discomfort to the patient.

Patient 4–5: Vocal Function
Analysis/Vocal Tremor

The patient was an energetic, self-referred, 80-year-old female who had recently noticed changes in her speaking voice. She described feeling a "loss of control" when speaking. This troubled her greatly, although family members and friends could not detect a change.

Laryngeal examination showed slight vocal fold bowing and mild atrophic changes consistent with the aging process. The impression was presbylaryngis and the patient was referred for voice evaluation.

During instrumental voice testing, the patient was asked to maximally sustain the vowel /a/ and maximally increase and decrease pitch and loudness. The results revealed a mild vocal tremor that was barely perceptible during conversation, and maximally evident during phonation at a low f_0 range in modal register. The sound spectrum showed regular and predictable oscillations in the acoustic waveform occurring at a rate of five times per second (Figure 4–17). These oscillations corresponded to changes in the phonatory flow signals obtained during aerodynamic testing. Steady airflow rates measured during sustained voiceless fricative sounds /s/; /f/ confirmed that the respiratory system, tongue, and lips were not involved in the tremor.

Following evaluation, both the videostroboscopic sample and the graphic output from the vocal function tests were utilized to help explain the nature of the voice disorder to the patient and her family. Although she decided not to pursue further evaluation or treatment, she commented at the conclusion of the counseling session that she felt relieved just understanding the cause and nature of her problems.

Laryngeal Electromyography (LEMG)

LEMG is a specialized procedure, not routinely performed, that offers unique diagnostic information on the electrical activity of laryngeal muscles. LEMG can be used to detect both normal and abnormal activity, assess degree of nerve damage in patients with vocal cord palsy, and provide prognostic indicators for the management of vocal cord paralysis (Blair, Berry, & Briant, 1978).

Although laryngeal electrodiagnosis can be a useful clinical tool in assessing a wide variety of vocal abnormalities, the procedure has been particularly beneficial in the assessment of traumatic injury to the larynx, laryngeal dystonias, and laryngeal paralysis. In cases of traumatic injury to the larynx, vocal fold immobility might be a result of either laryngeal paralysis or fixation of the arytenoid cartilage. The results of EMG testing aid in determining the cause of impaired mobility. In patients with laryngeal dystonias such as spasmodic dysphonia, the results can assist in identifying early manifestations of the disorder and help in determining the optimal injection site for botulinum toxin (Figure 4–18). In cases of laryngeal paralysis, EMG testing can aid in establishing evidence of reinnervation activity and assist in predicting future return of function. Because many of the treatments for laryngeal paralysis are not reversible, the EMG results may influence treatment choice and timing.

In most EMG diagnostic clinics, the muscle activity of the thyroarytenoid (innervated by recurrent laryngeal nerves) and cricothyroid muscles (innervated by superior laryngeal nerves) are studied bilaterally using either monopolar or concentric nee-

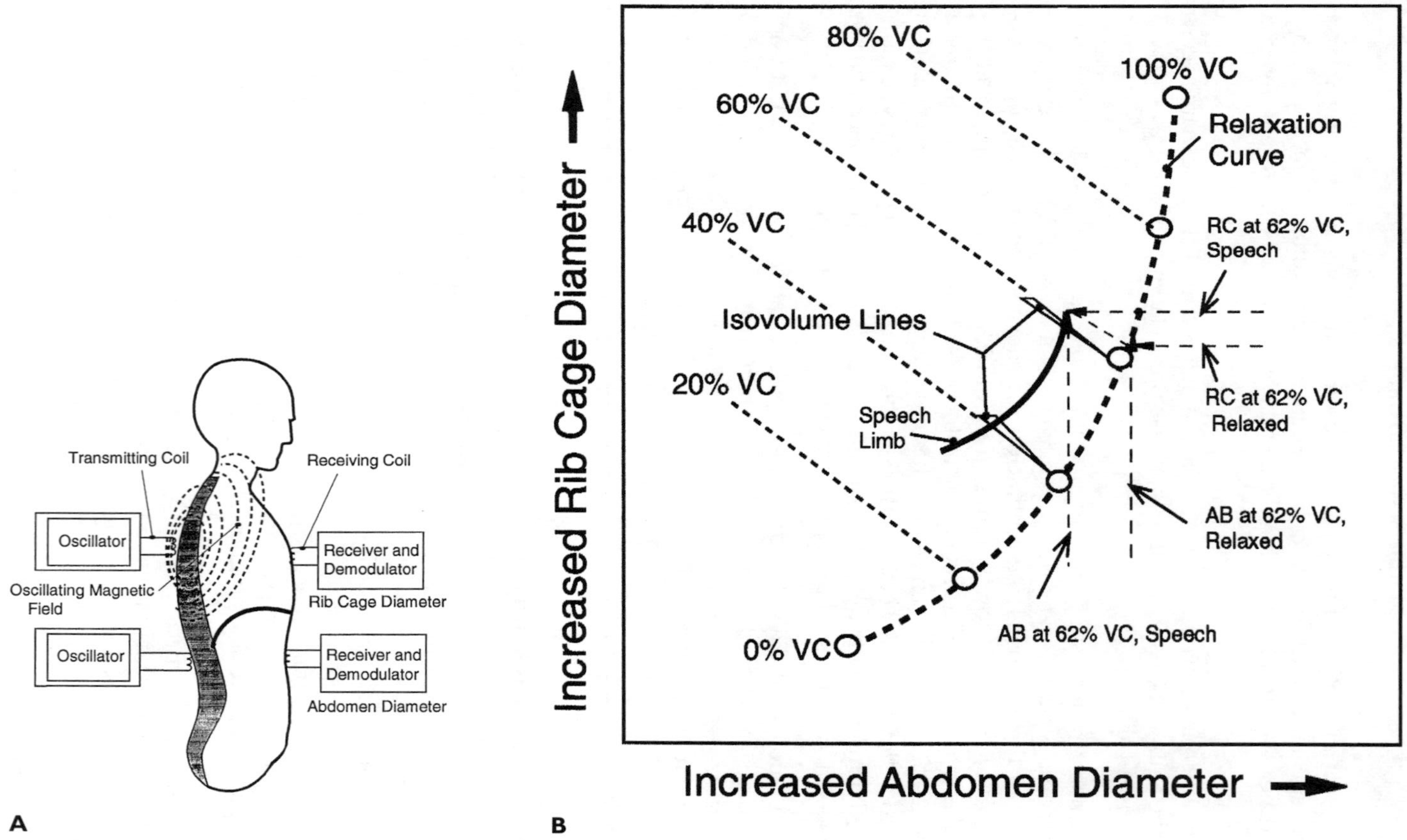

Figure 4–16. Kinematic measurement of speech-breathing patterns. **A.** Hardware design for measuring kinematics of the chest wall with magnetometers. **B.** Idealized motion-motion graph, showing abdominal and rib-cage movements (speech limb) relative to an individual's relaxation curve profile. (Reprinted with permission from M. D. Morrison & L. A. Rammage et al., 1994, p. 170–171. *The management of voice disorders.* London: Chapman & Hall Medical/San Diego: Singular Publishing Group, Inc.)

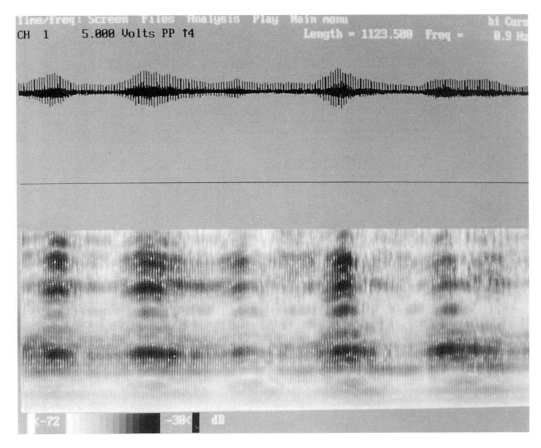

Figure 4–17. Sound waveform (*upper*) and wide-band spectrogram (*lower*) demonstrating 5 Hz vocal tremor.

dle electrodes. Because special equipment and expertise, as well as more invasive procedures, are required to study the posterior cricoarytenoid (PCA) muscles, they are not routinely sampled.

The diagnostic LEMG procedure used most commonly in clinical settings involves percutaneous placement of electrodes into selected laryngeal muscles, with the patient awake in a comfortable, supine position. The physician, usually a specialist in neurology or rehabilitation medicine, begins by preparing the patient through proper positioning, placement of a reference electrode on the forehead, and injecting a topical anesthetic at the electrode insertion site.

As the needle pierces the skin, the electrode is directed toward the targeted muscle while the physician continuously monitors EMG activity to observe insertion activity and to identify correct electrode placement. Confirmation of correct placement is achieved through the use of various laryngeal maneuvers that involve different muscle groups. For example, since cricothyroid activity varies responsively with changes in pitch (e.g., diminished activity at low pitches and increased activity at high pitches), pitch changes are included in the cricothyroid protocol. The presence of appropriate changes in muscular activity on this and other cricothyroid-specific tasks confirm cricothyroid electrode placement.

Bless (1991a) identified six features of EMG tracings that help clinicians make diagnostic decisions: electrical silence, fibrillation potentials, high-amplitude potentials, polyphasic potentials, normal potentials but reduced in number, and normal potentials.

In general, the procedure takes 30 to 50

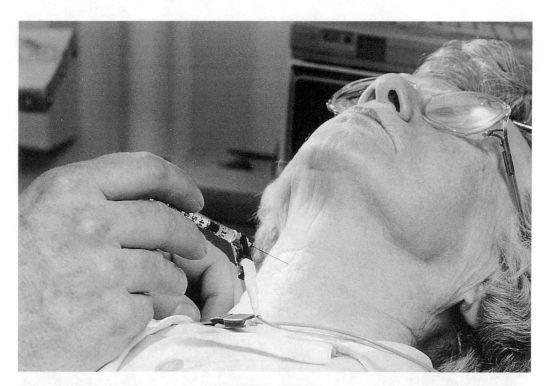

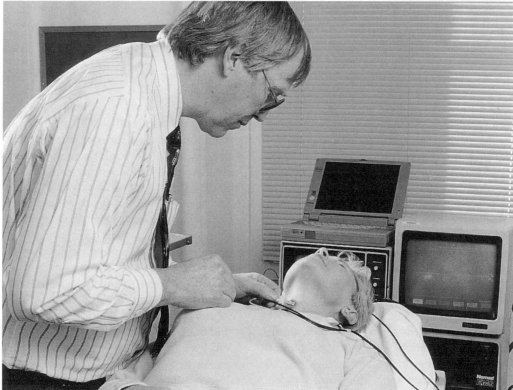

Figure 4–18. Laryngeal EMG procedure being used to guide the surgeon during an injection of botulinum toxin for focal laryngeal dystonia.

minutes. An additional observation time of approximately 30 minutes might be required prior to discharge. Although complications are rare, potential risks associated with LEMG testing include infection, bleeding, reaction to the anesthetic, and damage to adjacent structures (Luschei & Hoffman, 1991). Luschei and Hoffman identified several contraindications for percutaneous LEMG:

▶ Bleeding disorder (coagulopathy or use of coumadin or aspirin).

▶ Altered anatomy (from previous surgery, infections, or trauma) precluding percutaneous placement of the needle electrodes.
▶ Inability of the patient to cooperate (young children, adults with a psychiatric disorder or with severely compromised health).

Both with and without anesthetic, patients report mild to moderate temporary discomfort during the examination. One patient commented that the test made him feel like "an olive in a martini glass."

Patient 4–6: LEMG / Involuntary Muscular Activity

This 56-year-old school teacher presented with an 8-month history of voice changes. His initial symptom was uncontrollable pitch and voice breaks that occurred after he spoke just a few words. As he continued to speak, his effort level would increase and he found it necessary to force his words out. Onset of these difficulties had evolved slowly during the first 4 months and then his symptoms plateaued. He denied any obvious systemic or neurologic symptoms. The only medical problems he reported were high blood pressure and high cholesterol.

Both mirror examination and videostroboscopy revealed incomplete glottic closure with a slight glottal gap extending along the membranous length of the folds. Both vocal fold edges appeared slightly bowed and mildly atrophied with a possible furrow or sulcus of the left vocal fold edge.

Although the patient's physical symptoms were consistent with atrophic changes of the vocal folds, an EMG study was requested to rule out dystonic muscle activity. LEMG revealed involuntary muscle activity in both cricothyroid and thyroarytenoid muscles bilaterally. The problem was represented by muscle spasms leading to phonation breaks within speech phrases, and by involuntary muscle activity at rest (Figure 4–19). These findings appeared compatible with a laryngeal dystonia. They clearly established the need for further neurological evaluation.

Comprehensive neurological testing, including MRI and CT, was performed with equivocal results. A number of very "soft" findings (i.e., facial asymmetry) and questionable signs and symptoms referable to the left ponto-medullary junction (vascular thrombosis) were noted, but no active pathology was identified. When the patient returned to the Voice Clinic to discuss the diagnostic results, the voice care team recommended treatment with botulinum toxin since his voice problems appeared related to inappropriate muscular activity. He was subsequently treated with bilateral injections into the thyroarytenoid muscles using LEMG guidance. At his 1-month follow-up visit, he reported dramatic improvements in pitch control and voice quality, and more fluent speech in response to treatment .

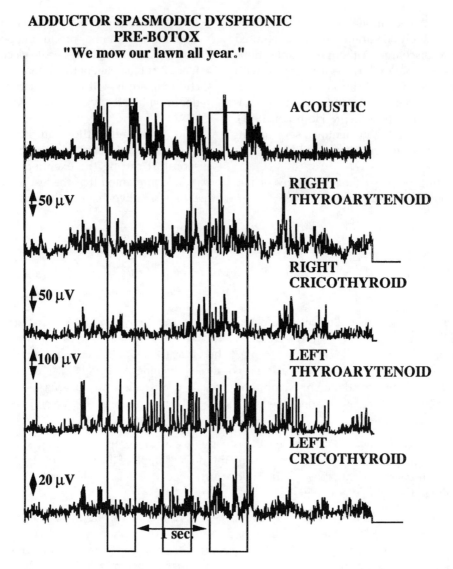

Figure 4–19. Intrinsic LEMG hooked wire recordings from a patient with adductor spasmodic dysphonia with speech breaks while saying the sentence: "We mow our lawn all year." The points in the speech with breaks are contained in rectangular boxes showing the coincident muscle spasms while the patient has a voice break.

ENSURING PROPER USE OF EQUIPMENT

According to B. F. Skinner, "Data speak—not men." This quotation aptly reflects the attitude held by many regarding the nature of instrumental evaluation. There is a common belief among those not intimately acquainted with the use of instruments that measurements produced by laboratory equipment are always consistent, objective, and reliable measures of performance. Not necessarily true! A number of variables, both technological and human, can threaten the reliability or validity of instrumental measures throughout the course of data collection, analysis, and interpretation.

Among the potential misuses and abuses of instrumentation are issues of equipment calibration, capacity and use, test selection, data acquisition and handling, test environment, and judges' abilities. Several guidelines for instrumentation use can assure the most valid and reliable measures, regardless of which array of instruments is used.

Equipment Calibration

Special care must be taken to ensure calibrated recordings, as faulty, inadequate, or changing calibration of equipment can invalidate clinical and research data. Aerodynamic instruments may be particularly vulnerable to faulty or changing calibration and may require daily or even more frequent recalibration. If inconsistency of data is present (e.g., values vary greatly from expected levels or from previously reported data), a calibration problem should be suspected.

Adequate Frequency/ Gain Response

One possible source of instrumental error is an inadequate frequency response range. If a patient's airflow rate, fundamental frequency, or vocal intensity level exceeds the limits of a particular instrument, a flattening effect will occur, yielding invalid measures. Airflow peaks can become flattened when the data acquisition and analysis system being used is incapable of assessing airflow rates beyond its capabilities (Figure 4–20).

Commonly observed problems attributable to this type of instrumental limitation are apparent in special populations such as the geriatric group, singers, children, and vocal fold paralysis patients. In geriatric patients, for example, mean airflow rates sometimes fall significantly below the normal and expected range (e.g., 30 cc/sec). Some singers also produce unusually low mean air flow rates (Peppard, 1990) and extraordinarily wide pitch ranges (e.g., <75 Hz >1000 Hz). Children can demonstrate either an extensive upper pitch range (e.g., >800 Hz) and/or incredibly loud productions (e.g., >100 dB), and some vocal fold paralysis patients have been known to generate extreme airflow rates (e.g., >800 cc/sec).

Proper Use of Equipment

Although misuse of equipment can occur for a number of reasons, the problem most often results from a failure to follow standardized procedures for a specific instrument. The clinician should never assume that all types of devices that measure the same parameter operate similarly.

For example, there are a variety of makes and models of sound level meters (SLM). Despite their commonalities, it is important to review the specific instructions provided with each instrument to obtain valid and reliable measures. Some instruments are to be held perpendicular to the sound source at a distance of 18 inches; others require the examiner to point the SLM directly at the sound source, less than 18 inches away. Failure to comply with the manufacturers' instructions can compromise test findings.

Appropriate Equipment Selection

Inappropriate equipment selection can occur if the clinician does not fully understand the purpose of an instrument. In these cases, data might mistakenly be interpreted to mean something they simply do not mean. In one case, a 5-year-old child with a cleft palate was being seen for a comprehensive assessment of velopharyngeal insufficiency, and a measure of nasal airflow was to be obtained. To make this measurement, the clinician selected the nasometer, a device that measures an acoustic ratio: acoustic ratio = nasal energy / (nasal energy + oral energy) × 100. The obtained value represents nasal resonance or "nasalance," according to the manufacturer.

Whereas a relationship likely exists between nasal flow rate (an *aerodynamic* measurement) and nasal resonance (an *acoustic* measurement), these parameters are *not* the same and must not be confused. Although the information obtained from the nasometer contributed valuable information to the assessment, the measurements were certainly not valid measures of nasal flow rate. Addi-

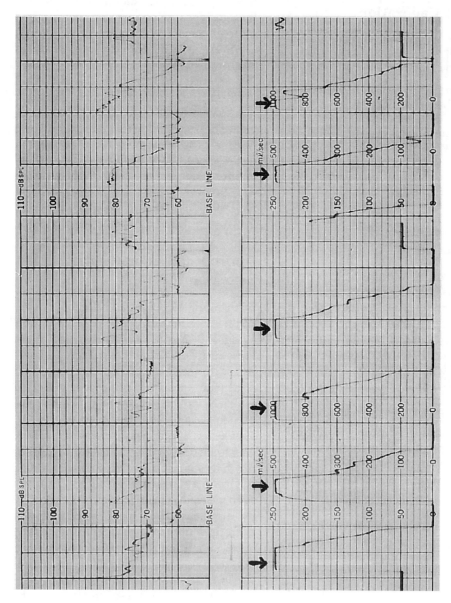

Figure 4–20. Aerodynamic recordings (mean flow rate-MFR on bottom graph) with peak-clipping. MFR is higher than 1000 ml/sec for this patient with recent unilateral vocal fold paralysis. Recording equipment measures only up to 1000 ml/sec therefore, the MFR signal is "flattened" and indeterminate for most of the phonation segments (arrows).

tional testing, using a pneumotachometer, flow transducer, and recording device or a rhinomanometer (which measures both nasal flow and pressure and calculates nasal resistance) would have been necessary to validly assess the targeted parameter.

Adequate/Appropriate Data Acquisition

It is the responsibility of the examiner, not the instrument, to establish test protocols, to provide instructions to the patient, to monitor the patient's behavior during testing, and to elicit optimal performance on maximum performance tasks. To achieve these ends, several suggestions are offered:

▶ Use standardized protocols that allow test/retest comparisons.
▶ Watch the patient as well as the equipment during all instrumental testing. Failure to do so can result in measures obtained while the patient is holding a face mask incorrectly, leaning into the microphone, or adopting an atypical posture or breathing pattern in response to the testing situation.
▶ Monitor the sound of the voice and the instrumental reading continually to make sure that the task is being performed properly. If the patient needs to make a change in behavior, reinstruct or provide modeling to assist the patient in achieving the desired response.

One common example of this prevalent clinical problem is the patient who demonstrates a tendency to elevate habitual pitch during sustained vowel productions. This behavior can produce erroneous test results across several measures (e.g., videostroboscopic measures of vibratory patterns or mean phonatory flow rates) because judgments of glottic closure, muscosal wave, vibratory amplitude, and habitual pitch are to be sampled at normal pitch and loudness (NPNL); and phonatory patterns and flow rates vary with f_0.

▶ Provide standardized instructions and offer encouragement and/or coaching on maximum performance tasks. Bless and Hirano (1982) confirmed that an individual's performance can be improved on a maximum phonation task by providing clearly stated verbal instructions in combination with encouragement and coaching. After studying the effects of these strategies on a group of normal subjects performing a maximum phonation task, they concluded: "Instructions which specifically asked subjects to inhale and exhale maximally, and which encouraged them to keep going near the end of their phonation, yielded significantly longer phonation times than did the use of instructions asking the subject to say /a/ as long as they could."

The same principles apply to the various respiratory and phonatory tasks included in instrumental voice protocols, such as dynamic pitch range, loudness range, maximum phonation time, forced vital capacity, flow loop volumes, and laryngeal diadochokinesis. Motivating the patient to perform optimally is a prerequisite to maximum performance tasks, and making pre- and post-treatment comparisons.

▶ Establish baseline stability by repeating tasks at least three times. Baseline instability can be due to changes in the examiner, the instrument, the patient, or an interaction of all three. Efficacious treatment planning requires that a stable baseline be established prior to intervention (see Chapter 6). A number of authors, including Sawashima (1966) and Bless and Hirano (1982), have addressed the question of how many trials are needed to make valid clinical comparisons. Most investigators agree that the use of three trials, with appropriate instructions, is sufficient to ensure a relatively high degree of reliability.

Appropriate Analysis Samples

Identifying and excluding inferior or inadequate analysis samples falls within the domain of the examiner, for no instrument can effectively distinguish between intended and actual human productions. In the case of a dysarthric speaker, for example, an intended sequence of /papapapapa/ might be executed motorically as /paʲ aʲ paʲ aʲ/. If the purpose of the task is to obtain a measure of mean intra-oral breath pressure, then the utterance must be repeated to acquire an adequate number of appropriate tokens for analysis. Failure to exclude syllables that do not contain the needed plosive /p/ would result in inaccurate intra-oral pressure values.

In other words, a co-dependency exists between the examiner and the instrument. A sophisticated instrumental system might be capable of producing simultaneous data on the audio signal, intra-oral air pressure, mandibular force, labial force, and lingual force. Nevertheless, it is the examiner who must decide the acceptability or unacceptability of a specific utterance.

Proper Testing Environment or Conditions

A number of environmental factors can adversely impact on a patient's performance during evaluation unless special attention is paid to the testing environment. To begin, a quiet test environment is essential for acoustic analysis. Both on-line direct analysis and the creation of high-quality acoustic recordings require a sound-treated space. The presence of ambient background noise can elicit atypical productions (e.g., Lombard effect) and render acoustic samples unsuitable for analysis.

A second consideration is that a vocal function laboratory filled with "high tech" equipment and instrumentation can be an intimidating or even frightening environment for many patients, especially young children. Efforts should be made to lessen the appearance of sterility and austerity in the instrumental voice laboratory and reduce distractions that might interfere with testing (see Chapter 7).

Third, many hospital and clinical settings (especially universities or teaching centers) are notorious for having large numbers of practitioners involved in the assessment process. Medical students, speech pathology interns, otolaryngology residents, a staff otolaryngologist, a staff speech pathologist, and other members of the voice care team might all be interested in observing the instrumental protocol. Although a few patients (usually performers) actually enjoy and thrive on such attention, the majority of patients feel uncomfortable with an "audience." Limiting or eliminating extraneous observers might be crucial to a successful and valid evaluation.

Judges' Competence

Despite the increased objectivity gained through instrumental evaluation, the process remains inherently subjective when humans are asked to make judgments or ratings on auditory or visual parameters of voice. Human instrumentation errors are most likely to occur when judges are insufficiently trained, inexperienced, or unobservant. The subjective ratings made during videostroboscopic analysis exemplify the situation. Clinicians must rate vibratory characteristics such as glottic closure, symmetry, periodicity, amplitude, and mucosal wave on the basis of their knowledge of normal structure and function, the mechanics of phonation, and the pathological effects of dysfunction and disease. Consequently, varying degrees of intra- and interjudge reliability might be evident, based on the experience and competencies of the examiner.

STRENGTHENING DATA INTERPRETATION

The potential contributions of instrumental analyses are actualized only in the hands of a skilled professional who interprets the data within an appropriate and meaningful context. It is the humans behind the machines who are ultimately responsible for data interpretation.

When interpreting test results, practitioners consider much more than just the numerical values or measurements obtained from instrumental testing. Their interpretative judgments must encompass a broader perspective that examines the role of each abnormal finding and explains its presence within the context of the total person. The isolated test measure constitutes only one part of a comprehensive test battery. As Ludlow (1982) points out, no single diagnostic technique (or measure) can be singled out as the most effective.

Although individual measurements have little, if any, interpretative value, clusters of measures obtained through the administration of a comprehensive, diagnostic battery can create a profile of the patient's vocal performance, enabling skilled professionals to make judgments regarding the etiology of the dysphonia. Based on test results, team members can define the severity of the disorder, draw conclusions about the pathogenesis of the problem, make comparisons to normative and group-disordered data, determine the need for further workup and generate treatment recommendations.

What test results cannot ensure is that the patient will necessarily perform in exactly the same way during subsequent testing. Despite the examiners' best efforts to elicit test results that are replicable—using standardized protocols, well-calibrated and suitable equipment, and appropriate procedures—two other primary factors related to patient variability may influence testing either favorably or unfavorably. These factors—the test conditions and/or environment; and the patient's internal state—are ever-present components of the interpretative totality.

All tests are to some extent reactive measures. That is, they have the potential for modifying the variables under study because they are not a part of the normal environment (Huck, Cormier, & Bounds, 1974). During instrumental testing, special care must be taken to reduce the reactive effects of procedures; in many cases, such effects are unavoidable. Factors such as patient discomfort during the examination, unnatural positioning or posturing during testing, the use of recording devices (e.g., video or audiotaping) or the placement of masks over the face or tubes in the mouth all create an abnormal environment. Consequently, in both interpreting and reporting test results, clinicians must, at the very least, be cognizant of these potential test artifacts.

Likewise, the patient's internal state can potentially alter test results. Factors such as the person's health on the day of the assessment, energy level at the time of testing, the influence of any events or activities that might have preceded evaluation, the effects of medications, or the patient's mood, anxiety level, and willingness to undergo testing might all impact on performance.

For the voice specialist, recognition of these overt and covert characteristics of individual patients provides the ultimate medium for developing interpretations. Just as a photographic image suddenly appears before the photographer, so do representations of a pathological condition emerge before the practitioner when the sum of these interacting processes are used in evaluating voice production.

Thus, a working hypothesis has been established and the instrument-aided assessment of the pathology is completed. The voice care team can begin the process of designing a therapeutic protocol for the patient.

REFERENCES

Baer, T., Titze, I., & Yoshioka, H. (1983). Multiple simultaneous measures of vocal fold activity. In D. M. Bless & J. H. Abbs (Eds.), *Vocal fold physiology: Contemporary research and clinical issues.* San Diego: College-Hill Press.

Baken, R. J. (1987). *Clinical measurement of speech and voice.* Boston: College-Hill Press.

Blair, R. L., Berry, H., & Briant, T. D. R. (1978). Laryngeal electromyography techniques and application. *Otolaryngology Clinics of North America, 11*, 325–331.

Bless, D. M. (1991a). Assessment of laryngeal function. In C. N. Ford & D. M. Bless (Eds.), *Phonosurgery: Assessement and management of voice disorders* (pp. 95–122). New York: Raven Press.

Bless, D. M. (1991b). Measurement of vocal function. *Otolaryngology Clinics of North America, 24*, 1023–1033.

Bless, D. M. (1993, July). *Vocal function assessment.* Presentation at Phonosurgery Symposium, Madison, WI.

Bless, D. M., Biever, D. M., Campos, G., Glaze, L. E., & Peppard, R. C. (1989). Videostroboscopic, acoustic, and aerodynamic analysis of voice production in normal adults. *Proceedings of the Vocal Fold Physiology Conference*, Stockholm, Sweden.

Bless, D. M., & Hirano, M. (1982, November). *Verbal instructions: A critical variable in obtaining optimal performance for maximum phonation time.* Paper presented at the Annual Convention of the American Speech and Hearing Association.

Castelijns, J. A., Castelijns, J. A., Gerritsen, G. J., Kaiser, M. C., Valk, J., Van Zanten, T. E., Golding, R. G., Meyer, C. J., Van Hattum, L. H., Sprenger, M., Bezemer, P. D. (1988). Invasion of laryngeal cartilage by cancer: Comparison of CT and MR imaging. *Radiology, 166*, 199–206.

Childers, D., Naik, J., Lavar, J., Krishnamurthy, A., & Moore, G. P. (1983). Electroglottography, speech and ultra-high speed cinematography. In I. R. Titze & R. C. Scherer (Eds.), *Vocal fold physiology: Biomechanics, acoustics and phonatory control.* Denver: Denver Centre for the Performing Arts.

Colton, R. H., & Casper, J .K. (1990). *Understanding voice problems.* Baltimore: Williams & Wilkins.

Dromey, C., Stathopoulos, E. T., & Sapienza, C. M. (1992). Glottic airflow and electroglottographic measures of vocal function at multiple intensities. *Journal of Voice, 6*(1), 44–54.

Hertegard, S., Gauffin, J., & Karlsson, I. (1992). Physiological correlates of the inverse-filtered flow waveform. *Journal of Voice, 6*(3), 224–234.

Hirano, M. (1981). *Clinical examination of voice.* Wien/New York: Springer-Verlag.

Hixon, T. J., and Collaborators (1987). *Respiratory function in speech and song.* San Diego: College-Hill Press.

Hirano, M., & Bless, D. M. (1993). *Videostroboscopic examination of the larynx.* San Diego: Singular Publishing Group.

Holmberg, E., Hillman, R., & Perkell, J. (1988). Glottal airflow and transglottal air pressure measurements for male and female speakers in soft, normal, and loud voice. *Journal of the Acoustical Society of America, 84*(2), 511–529.

Huck, S. W., Cormier, W. H., & Bounds, W. G. (1974). *Reading statistics and research.* New York: Harper & Row.

Kent, R. D., & Read, C. (1992). *The acoustic analysis of speech.* San Diego: Singular Publishing Group.

Kent, R. D., Kent, J., & Rosenbek, J. (1987). Maximum performance tests of speech production. *Journal of Speech and Hearing Research, 52*, 367–387.

Lee, C. K., & Childers, D. G. (1991). Some acoustical, perceptual, and physiological aspects of vocal quality. In J. Gauffin & B. Hammarberg (Eds.), *Vocal fold physiology: Acoustic, perceptual, and physiological aspects of voice mechanisms* (pp. 233–242). San Diego: Singular Publishing Group.

Ludlow, C. L. (1982). Research needs for the assessment of phonation function. In C. L. Ludlow & M. O. Hart (Eds.), *Proceedings of the Conference on the Assessment of Vocal Pathology.* ASHA Reports #11.

Luschei, E. S., & Hoffman, H. (1991, June). Use of the electromyogram (EMG) as a diagnostic aid for voice disorders. *National Center for Voice and Speech Status and Progress Report.*

McWilliams, B. J., Morris, H. L., & Shelton, R. L. (1990). *Cleft palate speech* (2nd ed.). Philadelphia: B. C. Decker.

Morrison, M. D., & Rammage, L. A., with: Nichol, H., Pullan, B., May, P., & Salkeld, L. (1994) *The management of voice disorders.* London: Chapman & Hall Medical & San Diego: Singular Publishing Group.

Peppard, R. C. (1990). *Effects of selected vocal characteristics of female singers and non-singers.* Unpublished doctoral dissertation, University of Wisconsin-Madison.

Rammage, L. A. (1992). *Acoustic, aerodynamic and vibratory characteristics of phonation with variable posterior glottis postures.* Unpublished doctoral dissertation, University of Wisconsin-Madison.

Rothenberg, M. (1973). A new inverse-filtering technique for deriving the glottal flow waveform during voicing. *Journal of the Acoustical Society of America, 53*, 1632–1645.

Rothenberg, M. (1977). Measurement of airflow in speech. *Journal of Speech and Hearing Research, 20*, 155–176.

Rothenberg, M. (1981). Some relations between glottal air flow and vocal fold contact area. In

C. L. Ludlow & M. O. Hart (Eds.), Proceedings of the Conference on the Assessment of Vocal Pathology. *ASHA Reports, 11.*

Salmon, S. J., & Mount, K. H. (1991). *Alaryngeal speech rehabilitation: For clinicians by clinicians.* Austin, TX: Pro-Ed.

Sawashima, M. (1966). Measurements of phonation time. *Japanese Journal of Logopedics and Phoniatrics, 7,* 23–29.

Schaefer, S. D. (1991). The treatment of acute external laryngeal injuries. "State of the Art." *Archives of Otolaryngology—Head and Neck Surgery, 117,* 35-39.

Slavit, D. H. (1995). Role of the pulmonary laboratory in voice assessment. In J. S. Rubin, R. T. Sataloff, G. S. Korovin, & W. J. Gould (Eds.), *Diagnosis and treatment of voice disorders.* New York/Tokyo: Igaku-Shoin.

Smitheran, J. R., & Hixon, T. J. (1981). A clinical method for estimating laryngeal airway resistance during vowel production. *Journal of Speech and Hearing Disorders, 46,* 138–146.

Sodersten, M., & Lindestad, P-A. (1992). A comparison of vocal fold closure in rigid telescopic and flexible fiberscopic laryngostroboscopy. *Acta Otolaryngologica (Stockholm), 112,* 144–150.

Sundberg, J. (1987). *The science of the singing voice.* De Kalb: Northern Illinois University Press.

Teitler, N. (1992). *Examiner bias: Influence of patient history on perceptual ratings of videostroboscopy.* Unpublished master's thesis, University of Wisconsin–Madison.

Titze, I. R. (1990). Interpretation of the electroglottographic signal. *Journal of Voice, 4*(1), 1–9.

Titze, I. R. (1991). Phonation threshold pressure: A missing link in glottal aerodynamics. *Journal of the Acoustical Society of America, 90*(4), 2344(A).

Titze, I. R. (1991). Acoustic interpretation of the voice range profile (phonetogram). *National Center for Voice and Speech Status and Progress Report, 1.*

Verdolini-Marston, K., Titze, I., & Druker, D. (1990). Changes in phonation threshold pressure with induced conditions of hydration. *Journal of Voice, 4*(2), 142–151.

Walker-Batson, D., & Purdy, P. D. (1991). Structural and functional brain imaging in disorders of speech and motor control. In D. Vogel & M. P. Cannito (Eds.), *Treating disordered speech motor control: For clinicians by clinicians.* Austin, TX: Pro-Ed.

Weissman, M. D., & Curtin, H. D. (1995). The current approach to imaging the larynx. In J. S. Rubin, R. T. Sataloff, G. S. Korovin, & W. J. Gould (Eds.), *Diagnosis and treatment of voice disorders.* New York/Tokyo: Igaku-Shoin.

APPENDIX 4–1

University of Wisconsin
Stroboscopic Assessment of Voice

| Name _____ |
| Hospital ID# _____ |
| Date _____ |
| Complaint _____ |

Glottic Closure

	Complete	Posterior	Irregular	Spindle	Anterior	Hourglass	Incomplete

Supraglottic Activity	○ None	① Slight compression of ventricular folds	②	③	④	⑤ Dysphonia plica Ventricularis V Folds not visible

Abuse _____

Allergies _____
Arthritis _____
Aspiration _____
Esophageal reflux_____
Neurological _____

Vertical Level of VF Approximation	○ Glottic Plane	①	②	③	④	⑤ Off Plane

Psychological _____

Thyroid _____
Other health problems _____

Vocal Fold Edge	Left	○ Smooth Straight	①	②	③	④	⑤ Rough Irregular
	Right	○	①	②	③	④	⑤

Strobe Comments & Interpretations _____

Amplitude	Left	○ Normal	① Slightly Decreased	② Moderately Decreased	③ Severely Decreased	④ Barely Perceptible	⑤ No Visible Movement
	Right	○	①	②	③	④	⑤

Mucosal Wave	Left	○ Normal	① Slightly Decreased	② Moderately Decreased	③ Severely Decreased	④ Barely Perceptible	⑤ Absent
	Right	○	①	②	③	④	⑤

Non-vibrating Portion	Left	○ None	① 20%	② 40%	③ 60%	④ 80%	⑤ 100%
	Right	○	①	②	③	④	⑤

Aerodynamics_____
Flow_____Volume_____
Pressure _____

Acoustics _____
Frequency_____Intensity_____
Perceptual Quality _____
Pitch_____Loudness_____
Stridor_____Hoarseness_____
Breathiness _____
Recommendations _____

Phase Closure	-5	-4	-3	-2	-1	0	1	2	3	4	5
	Open Phase Predominates (Whisper Dysphonia)					Normal					Closed Phase Predominates (Glottal fry—extreme hyper-adduction

Phase Symmetry	○ regular	① irregular during end or begin tasks	② irregular during extremes pitch or loud	③ irregular during 50%+	④ generally irregular 75%+	⑤ always irregular

Regularity	○	①	②	③	④	⑤

APPENDIX 4–2

Sample Protocol for Video-Laryngostroboscopic Evaluation

A. WITH CONTINUOUS (OBSERVATION) LIGHT:

1. Observe *normal respiration* for symmetry; abduction; extraneous movements; lesions/irregularities on vocal fold edges; minimum 20 sec.
2. *Laryngeal DDK:* /h i h i h i h i h i h i . . ./ minimum 3 trials (DDK averaged over minimum 10 repetitions)
3. Observe abduction during *forced inhalation* (3 trials)
4. Observe *cough:* adduction; changes in larynx position
5. Observe glottis/larynx during phonation /i/ : modal register note vocal fold, supraglottic, and larynx postures; minimum 5 sec.
6. Slow glissandos (pitch sweeps) upward; downward. Note postures during pitch changes

B. WITH STROBOSCOPIC (FLASHING) LIGHT:

Set strobe to flash 2–3 Hz off f_0:

1. Observe vibratory patterns at average typical speaking pitch (modal register) on sustained /i/ minimum 3 trials for minimum 5 sec. each for ratings of: glottic/supraglottic closure patterns; vertical level of vocal fold approximation; amplitude of vibration; mucosal wave; nonvibrating portions; phase closure & symmetry
2. Observe vibratory patterns; glottic and supraglottic postures and larynx position at high and low pitches
3. Observe vibratory patterns; glottic and supraglottic postures and larynx position at loud and soft intensities
4. Observe vibratory patterns; glottic and supraglottic postures and larynx position during slow glissandos; note register transitions
5. Observe vibratory patterns; glottic and supraglottic postures and larynx position during stimulability probes: (cough; sigh; inhalation phonation; gentle onset; pitch changes; nasalizing)

Set strobe to flash at f_0 (phase-locked):

6. Observe vibratory patterns: for regularity (periodicity) /i/ typical pitch, modal register, minimum 5 seconds
7. Observe vibratory patterns: (regularity) at high and low pitches; loud and soft intensities; stimulability probes

C. WITH TRANSNASAL FIBEROPTICS:

1. Stop above velo-pharynx to observe V/P closure during vocal and nonvocal tasks (closure patterns/symmetry/degree):
   sustained vowels: /a/; /i/; /o/; /u/
   sustained fricatives: /s/; /f/ VS nasals: /m/; /n/
   syllable repetition: /pipipi . . . /; /sisisi . . . /
   counting: *50–70; 80–100*
   spontaneous speech: monologue; name; occupation; hobbies
2. Stop above epiglottis to view larynx and glottis for postures/closure patterns during connected speech:
   Spontaneous speech: monologue; question responses
   Standard sentence repetition for maximum glottic view:
   "Please keep three pieces of cheese for me" (3 trials)
3. Observe larynx and glottis for postures/closure patterns:
   glissandos; and repertoire singing, where applicable
4. Observe larynx and glottis during stimulability probes
5. During sustained /i/, move scope closer to vocal folds to observe vibratory patterns with stroboscopic light; moving scope out of larynx between phonation segments to minimize contact/gagging

APPENDIX 4–3

Sample Protocol for Acoustic and Prosodic Assessment

A. FUNDAMENTAL FREQUENCY PARAMETERS

Physiological Range   Low f_0: _____ Hz.; register:
(maximum performance;
min 3 trials)   High f_0: _____ Hz.; register:

Register Breaks/Transitions (f_0): _____; _____; _____

f_0 Flexibility/Continuity (comments): _____

Tessitura: S A T B   Singing Range/Registers: _____

Mean Speaking f_0*: _____ Hz; typical speaking register: _____

Speaking f_0 Range*:   Low: _____ Hz.; register:
(*sampled from 3 minute
min. spontaneous speech): High: _____ Hz.; register:

f_0 of nonverbal sounds: *"um hum"*: _____ Hz.; *"hm!"* _____ Hz.

                           laughing: _____ Hz.; coughing: _____ Hz.

Difference: spontaneous sounds VS mean speaking f_0: _____ Hz.

---

register codes: M = modal; F = falsetto; G = glottal fry; O = other
tessitura codes: S = soprano; A = alto; T = tenor; B = baritone/bass

---

B. INTENSITY PARAMETERS

Physiological Range   Low */a/*: _____ dB SPL
(maximum performance;
min 3 trials)   High *"Hey!"*: _____ dB SPL

Gradual Intensity Changes: < (cresc.): Low: _____ ; High: _____

(tasks: */a/*; counting)   > (dim.): High: _____ ; Low: _____

Maximum Intensity of Cough/Forced Adduction: _____ db SPL

Typical Speaking Intensity: Mean: _____ dB SPL

                             Range: _____ dB SPL - _____ dB SPL

Appropriateness/Adequacy of Speaking Intensity/Variability: _____

f_0/Intensity interdependence? (describe): _____

C. RATE/DURATION PARAMETERS

Sustained Phonation: */a/*: _____ sec.; */m/*: _____ sec.
(maximum performance;
best of min. 3)   *s/z ratio:* _____

Connected speech: Maximum Phrase Length: Serials: _____ sec.

(counting rate = 3 numbers/sec.)   Highest number: _____

Average Speaking Phrase Length: _____ sylls.; _____ sec.

Vocal DDK: */i/* : _____ (rep./sec.); */hi/* : _____ (rep./sec.)
(maximum performance; min. 10 sec. sample; best of min. 3 trials)

Typical Rate of Speech: _____ syls./sec; _____ words/min.

Prosody: Speaking Rate: *Normal* or *Fast* or *Slow*

                Vocal Fluency: *Normal* or *Abnormal* (describe)**

**Average number of dysfluencies/minute: _____
(Measure Voice Break Factor in D.)

Sound/Syllable Duration: *Normal* or *Abnormal* (describe)

Inflection: *Normal* or *Flat* or *Exaggerated*

Stress Pattern: *Normal* or *Reduced* or *Exaggerated*

Voice Onset Times: *Normal* or *Abnormal* (describe in D.)

Phrasing: *Normal* or *Long* or *Short* and/or *Agrammatical*

D. SPECTRAL-ACOUSTIC PARAMETERS

Signal-to-Noise Ratio (SNR):   */a/*: _____ dB; */o/*: _____ dB

SNR in phrase *"We will all go away"*: */a/*: _____ dB; */o/*: _____ dB

Perturbation Measures (e.g., Jitter/Shimmer):

VOT (if *Abnormal* in C.) Measure:

   VOT (msec) from wide-band (300 Hz) spectrogram:

   (*"Pay   him   sixty   cents   for   a   cup   of   hot   coffee"*)

   _____; ____; ____; ____; _____; _____; ____; _____

Voice Break Factor (VBF): _____ voice breaks/minute

APPENDIX 4–4

Sample Protocol for Aerodynamic Assessment of Voice Function

A. NONVOCAL RESPIRATORY FUNCTION:

1. **Forced Vital Capacity Measure:** minimum 3 trials of forced exhalation after forced inhalation, measure volume units with spirometer or pneumotachograph and mouth tube; nares occluded. Largest volume = FVC

2. **Tidal Volumes:** minimum 60 seconds; relaxed, quiet breathing in upright sitting position; using spirometer or pneumotachograph with mouth tube (nares occluded) or face mask covering mouth and nose. TV = averaged volumes for successive cycles

B. PHONATORY FLOW RATES AND VOLUMES:

Use flow transducer with full or partial face mask (divided for separation of nasal flow/oral flow, where indicated). Make simultaneous measures of f_0 and intensity for all vocal/speech tasks. Control intra-task trials for f_0/intensity.

1. **Sustained vowels:** /a/; /i/ at typical pitch/loudness; minimum 3 trials. Calculate MFR for each vowel (cc/sec; ml/sec).

2. **Flow rates; sustained vowels:** /a/; /i/ at high and low pitches; loud and soft intensities (same as those used for laryngo-stroboscopic evaluation). Calculate MFRs for each vowel (cc/sec; ml/sec).

3. **Maximum phonation time; flow rates; phonatory volumes; MPTs on vowels:** /a/; /i/ typical pitch and loudness; train/cue to ensure maximum performance. MPT = best of min. 3 trials for each vowel.

4. **Glissandos (gradual, sweeping pitch changes) through entire range.** Train/cue to ensure maximum performance. Record MFR with simultaneous pitch changes. Minimum 3 trials.

5. **Continuous speech** (note potential masking effect; and face movement restrictions due to mask):

   Counting; Spontaneous speech: name; occupation; hobbies. Record MFRs during speech.
   Standard sentence for speaking MFRs with voiced segments only:

   Repeat 5 times, normal rate: *"We were away a year ago."*

6. **Stimulability probes.**

C. PHONATION PRESSURE AND RESISTANCE ESTIMATES:

Use pressure transducer with intraoral tube; flow transducer, and face mask (divded for nasal-oral flow separation if necessary)

1. *"Say /pœ pœ pœ . . . / at this speed* (model 1.5 syll/sec), *using your usual effort and loudness."* Obtain intraoral pressure measurement (sub-glottal pressure estimate) cm H_2O on /p/; MFR on /œ/. Glottal resistance = pressure/flow.

   Average over minimum 3 trials, minimum 10 repetitions each trial.

PHONATION THRESHOLD PRESSURE-PTP (use pressure transducer):

1. Patient training and patient production calibrating to produce /pœ pœ pœ . . . / repetitions (as above):

   a. **suprathreshold level** [the force or "effort" level (cm H_2O) just above minimum required for phonation]

   b. **subthreshold level** [the force or "effort" level (cm H_2O) just below minimum required for phonation]

    c. phonation threshold [minimum force or "effort" level (cm H_2O) required for phonation to occur]

2. Phonation threshold pressure PTP (cm H_2O):

Average over minimum 3 trials, minimum 20 repetitions each trial.

CHAPTER

5

ROLES, RELATIONSHIPS, AND INTERDISCIPLINARY REFERRALS

Changes in technology have effected changes in the roles of various voice care professionals. The role of speech pathologists in assessment and diagnosis has expanded in parallel with advancements in instrumental and behavioral management techniques. This development has caused otolaryngologists and other specialists to reassess their opportunities for maximizing patient care.

ROLES AND RELATIONSHIPS

The Otolaryngologist/Laryngologist

The otolaryngologist (ENT physician) functions as both a surgeon who is a specialist in head and neck surgery and a practitioner of medical therapy who evaluates and treats

patients in the clinical setting. This role involves diagnostic, counseling, pharmacological, and surgical aspects of care. The professional title, *laryngologist*, implies a particular specialization in disorders of the larynx and voice.

In the assessment of voice patients, the otolaryngologist obtains a history and then performs a visual inspection of the ears, nose, oral cavity, pharynx, and larynx. Visualization of the larynx is generally made with a laryngeal mirror and/or a nasolaryngoscope; some practitioners supplement the physical examination with a videostroboscopic study. If medical difficulties arise during the course of testing (e.g., laryngospasms or reactions to an anesthetic), these problems are usually managed by the laryngologist. Following comprehensive evaluation that includes assessment by other team members, the physician diagnoses and counsels the patient regarding the presence or absence of possible laryngeal pathologies (e.g., cancer, papilloma, or dermoid cyst).

Throughout the assessment and treatment process, the laryngologist functions as the quarterback for the voice care team by referring patients for needed collateral testing (e.g., chest x-ray, blood test, MRI, or pulmonary function studies) and by coordinating the results. Following the assessment, the laryngologist may continue to quarterback a patient's treatment regimen by prescribing medications, seeking further consults, or performing surgery.

As a head and neck surgeon, the otolaryngologist performs complicated laryngeal, nasal, and otologic procedures. Some surgeons also perform facial plastic surgeries, including cosmetic and reconstructive procedures.

Each of these roles requires specialized training and a thorough knowledge of the organs and physical structures in the head and neck. Although it is not common for otolaryngologists to become subspecialists in phonosurgery, this trend is becoming more common today.

Additional roles and responsibilities are assumed by laryngologists affiliated with university teaching hospitals. Aside from their daily commitments to patient care, these specialists are involved in the education of medical students, residents, and speech pathology interns. They also conduct research and provide community service. Finally, the professional role of otolaryngologists can become defined by their knowledge of current, state-of-the-art approaches to the assessment and treatment process. Leadership positions and dissemination of information are activities assumed by those with state-of-the-art knowledge. As advocates for voice care, laryngologists act as a resource to their otolaryngology colleagues to eliminate outdated treatment methods such as "stripping the vocal folds" for bilateral vocal fold nodules.

In general, the practice of otolaryngology necessitates space for exam rooms, a special procedure room, and of course, the operating room.

There is an increasing trend toward use of a free-standing surgical unit among private practitioners and an outpatient ambulatory unit in hospitals, to eliminate the need for overnight patient visits following minor surgery.

The basic armory of diagnostic and treatment instruments used or accessed by the otolaryngologist are generally available even in small, rural community hospitals. One major exception is the availability of a clinical voice laboratory. Until recently, vocal function laboratories were found almost exclusively in medical-surgical teaching hospitals or research laboratories. Today, they enhance voice care services in a variety of medical settings including individual and group otolaryngology practices, as well as hospital-based clinics. However, despite their increasing prevalence, state-of-the-art vocal function laboratories are not yet routinely accessible to the majority of otolaryngologists.

The Speech-Language Pathologist/Speech Pathologist

The traditional role of the medical speech-language pathologist has focused on providing diagnostic and therapy services to patients with a wide range of communication problems (e.g., aphasia, dysarthria, stuttering, cognitive communication deficits, dysphagia, and voice disorders). Although the needs of some medical centers can still be met through the services of a generalist—a speech-language pathologist who serves diverse populations—other facilities now require staff members to demonstrate expertise and skills in a specialty area. Subspecialization in voice disorders is gradually becoming the clinical standard of practice in medical settings. This change in the role of the speech-language pathologist is a natural and necessary consequence of rapid advancements in medical science and technology.

By definition, subspecialists are those who center their knowledge and skills on one organ or system of the body. Speech-language pathologists who subspecialize in voice disorders devote their clinical practice to the assessment and treatment of the phonatory system and the larynx. As practitioners they function as clinical experts in the physiology of vocal behavior, primarily as it relates to speech, singing, or other communicative activities. The professional title *speech pathologist* is used here to designate professionals with a specialized scope of practice. Although other subspecialists in the voice care team may focus on the integrity of the laryngeal structures, the speech pathologist's domain is that of normal and abnormal speech and vocal function. Consequently, they administer a battery of vocal function tests (e.g., videostroboscopy, electroglottography, aerodynamic and acoustic assessments) that allow them to observe, record, and analyze the patient's vocal behaviors methodically during speech and nonspeech activities. They then apply their knowledge and skills to interpret the findings to patients and their families. Speech pathologists' counseling sessions include a diagnosis of the patient's vocal pathology (e.g., muscular tension dysphonia, hypofunctional dysphonia, dysphonia related to vocal fold stiffness, improper use of pitch). Behavioral treatment sessions might involve vocal hygiene counseling, gastroesophageal reflux counseling, pre- and postoperative counseling and therapy, individual or group voice therapy, alaryngeal speech rehabilitation, and/or augmentative aid training (e.g., electronic communication devices and speech amplifiers). A more detailed discussion of voice therapy follows in Chapter 6.

Whereas speech pathologists remain premier diagnosticians and therapists, technological changes and specialized skills are bringing three major new facets to their roles: intraoperative monitoring, intraexamination behavioral management; and instrumental management. While some of these activities are performed cooperatively with the otolaryngologist or other medical staff, others remain autonomous.

Intraoperative Monitoring

During intraoperative monitoring, the speech pathologist and the laryngologist work as partners in the operating room. For example, during an Isshiki thyroplasty (Type 1) medialization procedure, the patient remains awake during the surgery so that voice can be carefully monitored while a silastic implant is inserted through a surgically created window in the thyroid cartilage. The speech pathologist aids the surgeon through visual and auditory monitoring of the patient.

Visually, the degree of glottic closure and the plane of the opposing vocal fold are carefully monitored while the implant is sized and inserted. When the patient phonates, perceptual characteristics of the voice are monitored as breathiness diminshes and voice quality and loudness improve. More sophisticated on-line acoustic analysis techniques may be used where indicated to indicate surgically induced voice changes. Through cooperative intraoperative monitoring techniques such as this, involving the surgeon, patient, and speech pathologist, optimal phonosurgical results can be obtained.

Behavioral Management/Laryngeal Imaging

Because speech pathologists have formal training in behavioral management approaches (e.g., relaxation therapies, behavioral conditioning), they are often successful in visualizing, through videostroboscopy, the larynges of patients who are otherwise extremely resistant to indirect visualization. This includes adult patients who are very gaggy, children (generally aged 7 or older), patients with psychological-emotional problems, or intellectually challenged individuals.

Whereas the expertise of the speech pathology examiner is no greater or lesser than that of the physician in manipulating the mirror or endoscope, the approach and time required for desensitization in a difficult-to-examine patient varies significantly. The extra time and effort required to explain the procedure, reduce distractions, relax or position the patient, and thus to instill a positive attitude toward testing may be more readily accommodated in the speech pathologist's scheduling practices.

Diagnostic Testing Using Videoendoscopy

Only recently has the value of diagnostic testing using videoendoscopy been fully recognized in voice care clinics. Many voice care teams now routinely make use of this method to assess the potential benefits of various phonosurgical and behavioral management techniques.

The method involves use of either a rigid or flexible transoral endoscope, connected to a video system to allow imaging and documentation of the larynx. Laryngeal and manual compression tests and/or diagnostic probe therapy techniques can be used to induce voice improvements during visualization.

The role of the speech pathologist is primary to the diagnostic therapy process. Most commonly, the speech pathologist conducts this type of stimulability testing at the end of the videostroboscopic evaluation. Both the speech pathologist and the laryngologist may assess the auditory perceptual and physiological changes that occur during probe therapy.

Marketing and Program Development

In this age of managed care there is always a need to market health care services to remain competitive in the medical "marketplace." This is one of the expanding roles of the clinical speech pathologist.

Furthermore, in medical settings where a clinical voice laboratory is nonexistent, the clinician may assume primary responsibility for establishing one by negotiating with the institution's administrators, heading various fundraising activities, defining the targeted clinical population, selecting equipment, specifiying space requirements, establishing liaisons with appropriate institutional engineers and setting up the clinical voice laboratory.

Numerous public relations efforts may be necessary to develop and market voice care services (e.g., brochures; in-service education), particularly if clinicians have administrative responsibilities associated with their positions.

Management of Laboratory Instrumentation

One of the most challenging responsibilities assumed by voice specialists is setting up and maintaining laboratory instrumentation. The successful ongoing operation of laboratory equipment requires some knowledge and background in the mechanics of instrumentation as well as problem-solving skills and contacts with key persons (e.g., vendors; in-house engineering staff).

Frequently, the speech pathologist operates as the initial problem-solver or laboratory manager. Without this ongoing management and technological support, the voice clinic laboratory can quickly become dysfunctional.

The Voice Coach and Other Specialists

For patients who are performers or professional speakers, the perspectives offered by voice and drama specialists strongly complement those of the laryngologist and speech pathologist. Whereas their assessment strategies may overlap those used by the speech pathologist, the voice or drama coach more thoroughly examines each individual's vocal technique when performing (e.g., singing, acting, public speaking). For both the singing and drama specialist, primary components of an evaluation include the case history interview, observation of vocal technique, and counseling. As vocal problems are identified, alternative techniques, approaches, or behaviors are suggested and practiced during the assessment so that the patient can experience kinesthetic and auditory changes with the assistance of the vocal consultant. Explanation, modeling, listening, and understanding are among the most powerful tools used by these specialists. As kindred spirits sharing their love of the "art," they also share an understanding of professional needs and demands faced by the professional voice user.

Although consultations sometimes occur in the medical facility, typically patients are seen by the vocal pedagogue specialist in the voice studio and/or in the patient's performance venue. Generally, equipment needs for the voice or singing coach/pedagogue are minimal and typically include a piano or keyboard for the singing pedagogue. Recently, however, some voice teachers have begun to use sophisticated instrumentation to enhance vocal instruction. In these instances, a special laboratory may be dedicated to the professional voice user or laboratory instrumentation may be shared among interdisciplinary groups to optimize resources.

Occasionally, the professional roles of team members overlap. Although some might consider any redundancy of professional roles to be a weakness, others view it as a strength. The case history interview exemplifies the situation. When a new patient is seen for an initial evaluation, it is customary for each professional to interview the patient briefly at the beginning of the assessment. Not only does this practice assist clinicians in establishing rapport with the patient, it enables each practitioner to probe more comprehensively into his or her own particular area of expertise. Because of their training and background, different professionals focus on different aspects of the voice problem. For example, the otolaryngologist may examine more thoroughly the medical history and use of medications, while the speech pathologist explores in-depth daily voice use and vocal demands, and the singing specialist investigates specific aspects of a singer's performance schedule and voice training.

Another advantage of overlapping professional roles relates to the potential for the interchange of responsibilities between equally qualified specialists. For instance, both the laryngologist and speech pathologist might have received formal training in videostroboscopic examination. However, one of them might be more experienced or proficient in performing the procedure or have more time allotted for desensitizing patients who are difficult to examine. As long as professional roles are maintained and respected, certain procedures and services can comfortably be interchanged between team members.

Regardless of how a particular voice team chooses to divide or overlap certain responsibilities, all team members play key roles in the patients' care. Just as their collaboration is essential, so are their independent roles.

In summary, voice care can be considered a team effort, with each member bringing a unique perspective, knowledge base, and skill to the diagnosis and care of its patients. Experts from certain specialty areas are most likely to be involved on either a collaborative or consultative basis: Allergy and Clinical Immunology, Audiology, Dentistry, Endocrinology, Gastroenterology, Geriatrics, Human Oncology, Music, Neurology, Nursing, Pediatrics, Psychiatry, Psychology, Pulmonary Medicine, Rehabilitation Medicine, Rheumatology, and Theatre and Drama. They form the core of interdisciplinary voice care services.

Patient 5–1: Interprofessional Consultation—Conversion Disorder

A 78-year-old woman returned to her laryngologist complaining of hoarseness, laryngeal pain, and a sensation of a "lump in the throat" on the left side. This was the patient's third such episode of these symptoms, which were now presumed to be psychogenic, because the two preceding episodes had suddenly and completely resolved following direct microlaryngoscopy (DML) and exploratory surgery.

Although the physical findings had proven to be completely unremarkable on both previous occasions, the woman felt convinced that, during the operation, the surgeon had

continued

(continued)

removed the "lump" that was causing the problem, and that this was the explanation for her previous dramatic recoveries.

An interesting situation developed when family members contacted the otolaryngologist after her clinic visit, adamantly insisting that he perform a DML once more to help restore her voice. They argued that she was becoming increasingly depressed because of her inabilities to communicate, and that she refused to see a psychiatrist.

The dilemma here is clear, but the solution is not. Should the surgeon agree to perform a pseudosurgical procedure to help the patient regain her voice? Should symptomatic voice therapy be implemented while ongoing efforts are made to get the woman psychological help? Should the surgery be performed under the condition that she agree to see a psychiatrist?

These were some of the many questions posed by various members of a voice care team. As individuals from different disciplines, each professional might attempt to solve the problem a different way. As members of a team, they determined solutions through collaboration and coordinated care.

INTERDISCIPLINARY REFERRAL

In today's medical setting, interdisciplinary consultation is an intergral component of quality patient care. Requests for consultative services from specialists in the fields of Otolaryngology, Speech Pathology, Endocrinology, Psychiatry, Psychology, Pulmonary Medicine, Allergy, Neurology, Radiology, Gastroenterology, and Singing and Drama Pedagogy are not uncommon in the medical setting, given the complex nature of voice disorders and their various manifestations. Some basic procedural guidelines for referring patients to other specialties and for deciding when and to whom to refer voice patients can aid in maximizing the benefits of referral.

Basic Guidelines for Referring Patients

Once the decision has been made to refer a patient for consultation and/or treatment, the clinician must consider how to best proceed with the referral. Several basic guidelines can facilitate the process for all concerned.

Awareness of Available Resources

Although some voice patients may be able to return to their local communities for the necessary tests and/or treatment, others may need to be seen, at least initially, in a medical center where specialized expertise and equipment are available. For example, a patient suspected of having paradoxical vocal cord dysfunction (paradoxical motion of the vocal folds) may require comprehensive voice evaluation, including videoendoscopy, as well as pulmonary function studies (e.g., flow volume loops), and a short course of voice therapy involving biofeedback training. Knowing where voice specialty clinics are located within the community, state, or province can be invaluable to patients in need of specialized care.

Similarly, professional voice users, who would benefit from training for singing or public speaking, appreciate receiving, at the time of their assessment, the names of contact persons who provide these types of services. By keeping an updated listing of voice coaches, drama teachers, and instructors of public speaking, the clinician can assist the patient in following through with the recommendation. Providing resource lists of experts in other areas, such as those involved in biofeedback (relaxation) therapy, psychological counseling, and neuromuscular retraining can also be beneficial.

Patient Preparation

According to Schwab, Clemons, Valder, and Raulerson (1966), patients benefit more from consultation when they have been prepared by hearing a brief explanation of why a referral is being made, and by having an opportunity to ask questions. Misunderstandings and noncompliance often can be avoided by using this referral approach. This is particularly true of voice patients being referred for psychiatric or psychological evaluation. Without some type of rationale or explanation for the referral, patients may feel that the diagnosticians are really saying, "There's nothing wrong with your voice . . . the problem is all in your head." When offered brief, straightforward explanations, such as the ones below, the patient can better assume a participating role in the evaluative process.

> We [the voice team] are concerned about the stress that you're under, both at work and home, and as we've already discussed . . . there is probably a relationship between your voice problem and stress. To treat the problem in the best way possible, we're recommending that, in addition to voice therapy, you see a counselor, who can help you learn some stress management techniques. We'd be glad to give you the names of some experts in the area. Do you have any questions?

> We [the patient and examiners] seem to be in agreement about the probable causes of your voice problems. As you've mentioned, the voice strain occurs at times when you're feeling emotionally upset, and it is important to explore this relationship further to plan the best treatment for you. Because of this, we're recommending that you talk with our staff psychiatrist, who is an expert in this area. After you meet with her, we can talk again. Do you have any questions?

Consultant Preparation

It is important for the liaison consultant to understand the purpose of a referral prior to meeting with the patient. While this type of communication between the referrer and the consultant usually occurs via chart notes, personal contacts, or reports, occasionally a patient will appear in the consultant's office only to be asked, "Why are you here?" Negative feelings toward both the referral source and the consultant sometimes develop in these situations, particularly when the patient is already feeling reluctant about having the examination.

Furthermore, test findings may be compromised by inadequate communication. In the case of an electromyographic (EMG) study, for instance, it is critical that the examiner know specifically which muscles are to be assessed. For a patient with abductor spasmodic dysphonia, specific testing of the posterior cricoarytenoid muscles (PCAs) might not be performed if the consultant is simply given the diagnosis of spasmodic dysphonia, because the PCAs may not be routinely studied in all SD patients.

To facilitate the referral process, the consultant should be informed clearly of:

1. the purpose of the referral (e.g., requesting assistance in determining a diagnosis, seeking confirmation of a diagnosis, baselining information, a combination of the above),
2. the need for any special testing, and
3. identifying information about the referring clinician(s).

These measures make direct contact on the day of the consultation possible if required, and also improve postconsultative reporting.

Postconsult Patient Follow-Up

The trend toward subspecialization in health care has lead to a common scenario where an individual patient is sent to a variety of practitioners during the course of an evaluation. For example, as shown in Table 5–1, a

TABLE 5–1. An example of the assessment and consultative services provided to a patient scheduled for total laryngectomy.

Providers/Consultants	Activities
Otolaryngology	Head and neck examination, biopsy, patient and family counseling
Radiation Oncology	Medical consultation regarding possible benefits of radiation or chemotherapy treatments, head and neck examination, patient and family counseling
Speech Pathology	Voice and swallowing evaluations, patient and family counseling regarding post-op communication
Nursing	Pre-op home and self-care counseling
Cardiology	EKG, cardiac clearance for surgery
Pulmonary Medicine	Pulmonary function studies, pulmonary clearance for surgery
Radiology	Chest x-ray, CT/MRI scans, swallowing study
Clinical Laboratory	Blood tests
Anesthesiology	Anesthesia work-up
Social Services	Pre-op psychological/supportive counseling, preplanning for discharge placement/care
Clinical Nutrition	Pre-op feeding/nutritional counseling

patient with laryngeal cancer who is scheduled to undergo a total laryngectomy might come into contact with 11 or more different professions throughout the preoperative assessment and consultative process. With so many specialties involved in the patient's care, it is critical that the primary examiner or examiners keep the patient and his or her family informed regarding the test results, clinical findings, and recommendations, so that the patient doesn't get "lost" in the system.

For inpatients (e.g., those with laryngeal cancer), the otolaryngologist routinely functions as the primary coordinator for the patient's assessment and treatment programs. In the case of outpatients, various members of the voice care team may assume this responsibility, depending on the nature of the problem and the treatment plan.

For example, during the course of voice therapy it may become apparent to the speech pathologist that a patient would benefit from referral to a liaison consultant or therapist. In one instance, a trial attorney was referred to a psychologist for biofeedback training as an adjunctive measure to voice therapy because of excessive, generalized body ten-

sion. In this case, the speech pathologist coordinated the treatment program by following the patient's progress and responding to any questions or concerns regarding the referral.

What should ultimately be avoided in health care might be referred to as "serial referring," where one specialist refers to another. . . who refers to another . . . who refers to another—without diagnosis or resolution of the problem. Patients who present "difficult to diagnose disorders" may be at risk for this type of referral abuse, particularly when a team approach to voice care is not being used. Assuming (correctly) that the majority of voice disorders have two or more etiological bases can guide the voice care team in initiating appropriate referrrals and gathering cumulative diagnostic information from the various specialties to culminate in (a) differential diagnosis(es) and comprehensive management plan.

Referral to a Voice Care Team

Although traditional referral models have included assessments by a variety of disciplines, modern voice care philosophy emphasizes interdisciplinary collaboration between two or more subspecialty areas. The current approach to team care used in many voice specialty clinics bundles the services of otolaryngology and speech pathology to create a single, comprehensive voice evaluation package (Figure 5–1). Referrals for their assessment services come from a vari-

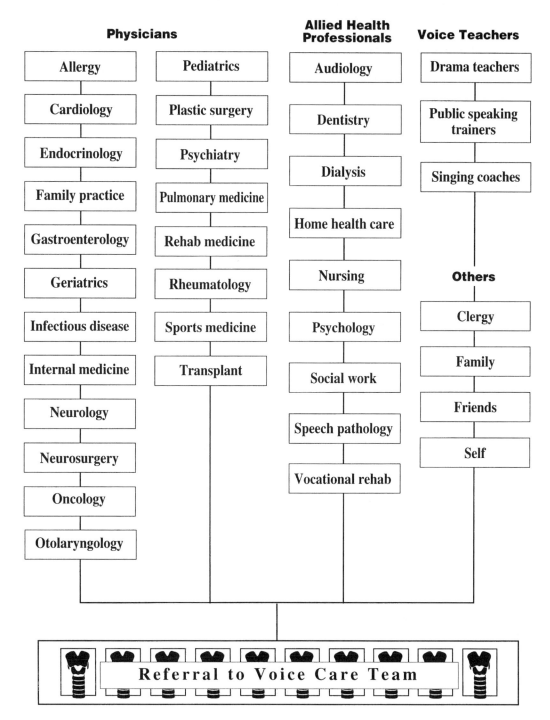

Figure 5–1. Referral to the Voice Care Team.

ety of sources, including other otolaryngologists and speech-language pathologists (generally those who are not members of an interdisciplinary voice team, and may not have access to the latest technological innovations), experts who offer voice instruction to professional voice users (either singing or drama training), physicians who see patients with systemic or multisystemic disorders, other medical or allied health professionals, nonmedical personnel or agencies, and family members, friends, or even the patient him/herself.

Even though it is highly desirable for other specialists such as neurolaryngologists and psychiatrists to participate fully in the evaluative and decision-making process, few voice care teams have immediate access to these professional services at the time of each patient evaluation. More commonly, these professionals tend to function as liaison consultants, meeting with selected patients on an "as needed" basis sometime after the initial clinic visit.

Following comprehensive evaluation by the voice care team, it may be necessary to refer the patient to one or more (sub)specialty areas for consultative or treatment services. The diagnostic diagrams which follow provide some suggested criteria for deciding when to refer patients with voice disorders to selected disciplines. Five subspecialty areas have been included, namely:

Endocrinology

Neurology

Psychiatry

Pulmonary Medicine

Speech Pathology

Although the suggested indications for referral may not always apply across patients and institutions, they can offer practitioners some general guidelines for referring to other disciplines.

Referral to Endocrinology

Endocrinology, a subspecialty of internal medicine, deals with the study of the endocrine glands. Endocrinologists, the specialists who diagnose and treat hormonal disorders, are most likely to be involved in the evaluation and/or management of patients suffering voice problems related to:

thyroid disease

gonadotrophin (sex hormone) deficiency

medication effects (androgens, corticosteroids)

pituitary or adrenal dysfunction

gender change

These are charted in Figure 5–2.

Thyroid Disease

Hypothyroidism (a condition in which the thyroid gland does not produce enough thyroid hormones to regulate the body's needs) may produce chronic edema of the vocal folds. Patients with an underactive thyroid may develop a hoarse, low-pitched speaking voice, secondary to laryngeal myxedema, as well as one or more of the systemic changes identified in Table 5–2.

In combination, these perceptual and physiological changes may lead the examiners to suspect an undiagnosed or untreated endocrine dysfunction, such as hypothyroidism. Referral to an endocrinologist is warranted in suspicious cases.

Occasionally, patients being treated for hypothyroidism may continue to present signs and symptoms of the disorder. If this occurs, patients are usually referred back to their physician to check the appropriateness of the dosage and type of medication, as well as patient compliance. Continuous monitoring of the patient's thyroid medication (levothyroxine sodium) is essential because different dosages may be needed at different times, and because some patients have a ten-

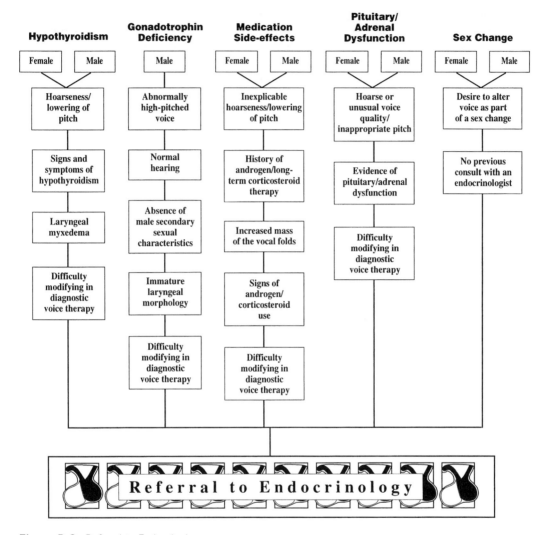

Figure 5–2. Referral to Endocrinology.

dency to self-administer drugs, that is, increase or decrease dosages without physician consultation. Even switching to a generic drug brand without checking with a physician beforehand can potentially compromise a patient's treatment program.

Gonadotrophin Deficiency

Gonadotrophins are the hormones made by the pituitary gland that begin the process of sexual development. In girls, these hormones stimulate the development of female secondary sexual characteristics by inducing the ovaries to produce estrogen and progesterone. In boys, testosterone, produced by the testes, is responsible for activating and maintaining male secondary sexual characteristics. Although slight differences in voice may be found in females with gonadotrophin deficiency when they are compared with their peers, the differences are negligible. In contrast, males with a sex hormone deficiency tend to demonstrate conspicuous vo-

TABLE 5–2. Signs and symptoms of hypothyroidism.

Psychological	Physical	Medical
Reduced concentration	Hair loss	Low serum T4/TSH levels
Reduced cognitive function	Face, ankle swelling	Goiter
Memory loss	Weight gain	Reduced GI, liver, kidney,
Depression	Dizziness, weakness	lung, heart functions
Anxiety	Headaches	Myxedema
Reduced mental development	Dry skin, nails, hair	Menstrual disturbances
	Cold sensitivity	Reproductive dysfunctions
	Fatigue, lethargy	Periorbital edema
	Reduced muscle strength	Reduced muscle tone
	Aches, pains, cramps	Anemia
	Anorexia	High cholesterol level
	Lip pallor	
	Constipation	
	Tongue swelling	
	Reduced perspiration	
	Heart palpitations	
	Dyspnea	
	Slow, dysrhythmic speech	
	Hoarseness, lowered pitch	
	Hearing loss	

cal symptomotology. As postpubescent young adults who have failed to experience the natural change in voice that occurs during adolescence, they present an immature laryngeal morphology and consequent abnormally high-pitched voices (which can fall either at the upper end of the chest register or in the falsetto range). Unlike young males with normal laryngeal structures who continue to speak using mutational falsetto, these individuals are nonresponsive to behavioral therapy. Another way in which they differ from their mutational falsetto counterparts involves their delay in developing typical male secondary sexual characteristics, such as facial hair, increased muscle mass, and masculine body shape and height.

Although this condition is rare, males suspected of having a gonadotrophin deficiency need to be referred for endocrinologic consultation. Diagnosed problems can be effectively managed with hormone replacement therapy.

Medication Effects

Changes in the female speaking voice may be related to androgen or androgen combination therapies (e.g., methyl testosterone, fluoxymesterone, testosterone cypionate, testosterone enanthate, testosterone pellets, esterified estrogens, conjugated estrogens, estradiol cypionate, estradiol pellets). The use of endocrine drugs, which may be prescribed to treat a variety of gynecologic disorders including endometriosis, breast cancer, and menopause, generally affect the larynx by increasing the size and mass of the vocal folds (Colton & Casper, 1990; Damste, 1964, 1967). Similarly, corticosteroids, often used as part of a treatment program for a number of different diseases or conditions such as arthritis, asthma, and severe allergies or skin problems, can potentially produce hormonally induced voice changes. With long-term usage, either males or females may experience alterations in voice (e.g., hoarseness, lowering of pitch) in addition to the other possible side effects. (*Note:* In some patients, prolonged corticosteroid usage may indirectly contribute to hoarseness by aggravating gastrointestinal problems and gastroesophageal reflux.)

The endocrinologist is one of several physicians who may be involved in administering a patient's drug therapy program. If the use of a particular medication appears to be irritating a preexisting condition (e.g., gastrointestinal problems) or producing side effects that concern the patient (e.g., an irreversible lowering of vocal pitch secondary to the use of an androgen or androgen combination medication), consultation with an endocrine specialist is recommended to determine if an alternative therapy or reduced dosage can alleviate the problems.

Pituitary or Adrenal Dysfunction

Hyperpituitarism is a condition in which there is an excessive amount of the growth hormone (GH) produced by the pituitary gland. When chronic hyperpituitarism exists, disorders such as acromegaly may develop with accompanying abnormalities in growth patterns and voice. Patients with acromegaly typically present a hoarse or unusual voice quality (secondary to laryngeal hypertrophy) as well as enlargement of the hands and feet, atypical facial features, and a variety of other signs and symptoms that are consistent with the disorder.

The excessive production of cortisol, due either to adrenal and/or pituitary dysfunction, can also produce voice differences. Cushing's syndrome, a disease characterized by truncal obesity, muscular weakness, moon facies, and a coarsening or deepening of the voice, may be due to an overproduction of the hormone adrenocorticotropin (ACTH).

In evaluating patients with either type of hormonal dysfunction, clinicians counsel their patients regarding the suspected cause of the dysphonia and encourage follow-up with an endocrinologist, should further counseling, evaluation, and/or treatment appear necessary. However, since these patients have the same chance of developing an independent vocal pathology as other persons of their age and sex, differential diagnosis is critical.

Gender Change

Patients planning a change in sex are routinely given hormonal treatments prior to undergoing surgery. However, many patients who are just beginning the inquiry process seek voice evaluation as an initial or early step toward sex change because they are concerned about developing a speaking voice that will be compatible with their new identity. Because of this, it is not uncommon for the otolaryngologist and/or the speech pathologist to be among the first professionals evaluating a patient who is considering sex change.

For these individuals, a referral to endocrinology is often the next step in the series to follow. If the services of a gender dysphoria team are available, counseling regarding hormonal treatments will be provided by one of the team members.

Referral to Neurology

The neurologist is a physician who specializes in diseases or conditions that affect the nervous system. Because voice and swallowing problems commonly coexist with neurological disorders, the services provided by the neurologist are an essential component of the total evaluation/management package in voice patients with disorders of neurologic origin.

The most common disorders referred for neurological consultation are outlined in Figure 5–3. Included are vocal aberrations associated with:

dysarthria

apraxia

essential voice tremor

laryngeal dystonia

idiopathic vocal fold paralysis

Tourette syndrome and other tic disorders

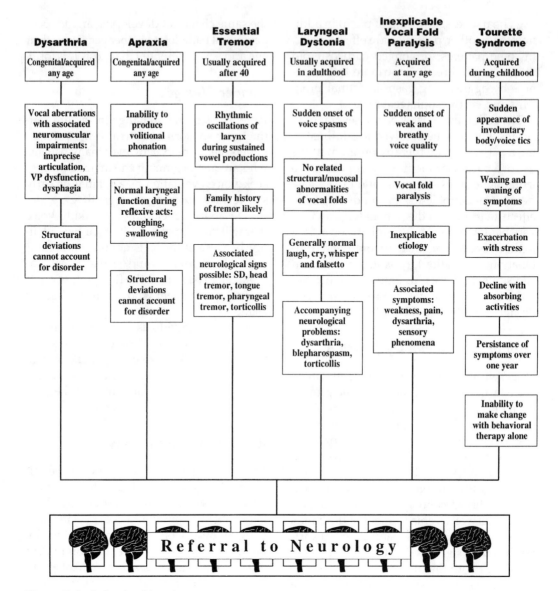

Dysarthria	Apraxia	Essential Tremor	Laryngeal Dystonia	Inexplicable Vocal Fold Paralysis	Tourette Syndrome
Congenital/acquired any age	Congenital/acquired any age	Usually acquired after 40	Usually acquired in adulthood	Acquired at any age	Acquired during childhood
Vocal aberrations with associated neuromuscular impairments: imprecise articulation, VP dysfunction, dysphagia	Inability to produce volitional phonation	Rhythmic oscillations of larynx during sustained vowel productions	Sudden onset of voice spasms	Sudden onset of weak and breathy voice quality	Sudden appearance of involuntary body/voice tics
Structural deviations cannot account for disorder	Normal laryngeal function during reflexive acts: coughing, swallowing	Family history of tremor likely	No related structural/mucosal abnormalities of vocal folds	Vocal fold paralysis	Waxing and waning of symptoms
	Structural deviations cannot account for disorder	Associated neurological signs possible: SD, head tremor, tongue tremor, pharyngeal tremor, torticollis	Generally normal laugh, cry, whisper and falsetto	Inexplicable etiology	Exacerbation with stress
			Accompanying neurological problems: dysarthria, blepharospasm, torticollis	Associated symptoms: weakness, pain, dysarthria, sensory phenomena	Decline with absorbing activities
					Persistence of symptoms over one year
					Inability to make change with behavioral therapy alone

Referral to Neurology

Figure 5–3. Referral to Neurology.

Dysarthria

In their text *Clinical Management of Dysarthric Speakers*, Yorkston, Beukelman, and Bell (1988) discuss associated signs and symptoms of the congenital dysarthrias (e.g., cerebral palsy, Moebius syndrome), the adult-onset nonprogressive dysarthrias (e.g., cardiovascular accident [CVA], traumatic brain injury), and the degenerative dysarthrias (e.g., amyotrophic lateral sclerosis [ALS],

Parkinson's disease, progressive supranuclear palsy, Huntington's disease, Wilson's disease, Friedrich's ataxia, multiple sclerosis [MS], myasthenia gravis, dystonia). While individual types of dysarthria present varying degrees of laryngeal involvement, phonation is typically disrupted, to some extent, in all dysarthric speakers.

Most commonly, it is the neurologist who refers dysarthric patients to other specialties for assessment following neurological evaluation. Sometimes, however, patients first notice problems with their speech, voice, or swallowing and subsequently seek assistance from other professionals, such as the otolaryngologist or the speech pathologist. Because of this, clinicians must be familiar with early manifestations of neurological disease, and refer suspicous cases on for neurological consultation.

Figure 5–3 shows a basic profile for the patient presenting dysarthria. Depending upon the nature of the disorder, the onset may occur either congenitally or be acquired after birth. There is typically involvement of more than one speech subsystem (e.g., hypernasal resonance, weak phonation, and imprecise articulation), and the dysfunctions cannot be related to structural deviations. Impairments of reflexive acts such as swallowing are common.

The traditional dysarthria classification scheme encompasses several specific types of dysarthria that frequently affect voice: benign essential tremors, focal dystonias, lower motor neuron paralyses, tic disorders, Parkinson's disease, other hyperkinetic and hypokinetic types of dysarthria, ataxia, and various progressive neurological diseases (e.g., ALS, MS) creating combinations of flaccid and spastic dysarthrias (Darley, Aronson, & Brown, 1975).

Essential Voice Tremor

The presence of tremulous phonation can signify neurological impairment, psychiatric disturbance, medication side effects, learned behaviors (e.g., singer's tremulo), or an emotional reaction to the test situation. Consequently, all patients with voice tremors are not referred for neurological evaluation.

For patients with regular, rhythmic movements or oscillations of the laryngeal structures, however, neurological consultation is advisable. Although the majority of these patients will be diagnosed by the neurologist with a benign essential voice tremor, often referred to as "familial tremor," it is important to rule out any other underlying pathophysiology (e.g., cerebellar degenera-

tive disease) and to evaluate the patient's suitability for the various available drug therapies (e.g., propranolol, phenobarbital, methazolamide) that may be used to alleviate tremorous laryngeal movements. Benign essential tremor can commence at any age, although middle-aged and older persons seem to be more susceptible than others (Koller, 1990). A familial history of some type of tremor is typical, as are associated neurological signs such as spasmodic torticolis, spasmodic dysphonia, head tremor, and tremors of the tongue and pharynx.

Currently, other than the use of systemic drugs such as those identified above, botulinum toxin and behavioral voice therapy are the only management options that have been found to provide any relief for patients with this central nervous system disorder.

Laryngeal Dystonia

Focal dystonias that are limited to the voice are generally recognized as the spasmodic dysphonias (SD). The presenting symptoms vary depending upon the positioning of the vocal folds during spasmodic activity (e.g., hyperadduction vs. hyperabduction).

Patients typically report a sudden onset of SD symptoms in adulthood, although some acquired pediatric cases have been seen. There is an absence of structural and mucosal abnormalities; other focal dystonias may or may not be present. Normal voice is often heard during spontaneous acts such as laughing and crying and when voice is produced in the falsetto register, as during singing in the upper pitch range. Although these patients may be modifiable during stimulability testing, they generally experience difficulty in maintaining their voice changes in behavioral therapy.

Since the primary purpose of a neurological consult is to rule out other diseases with similar vocal symptoms, SD patients presenting additional neurological problems (e.g., muscle weakness, dysphagia, dyspnea) or associated dystonic signs (e.g., blepharospasm, torticollis, writer's cramp) should be referred for neurological evaluation. Among the disorders that may be confused with SD are Parkinsonism, myoclonus, pseudobulbar palsy, tardive dyskinesia, cerebellar disorders, and MS (Woodson, Zwirmer, Murry, & Swensen, 1992).

Unexplained/Idiopathic Vocal Fold Paralysis

In patients with unexplainable vocal fold paralyses, a neurological examination should always be completed before considering diagnostic tests such as a CT scan, lumbar puncture, or electromyographic study. The purpose of the neurological consult is to obtain "a fuller evaluation of the integrity of the nervous system" (Tyler, 1988).

Patients with either unilateral or bilateral vocal fold paralysis, who exhibit related symptoms such as dysarthric speech or resonance features, muscle weakness, pain, sensory phenomena, or dysphagia are candidates for neurological assessment (Tyler, 1988). Those with a medical history of encephalitis or porphyria might also be considered for referral since vocal fold paralysis can be a sequla of these illnesses. Postencephalitic patients have sometimes experienced the onset of vocal fold paralysis after as long as 30 years.

Tourette Syndrome and Other Tic Disorders

Multiple tic disorders, such as Gilles de la Tourette syndrome (TS), generally include at least one vocal abnormality in addition to one or more involuntary motor behaviors. The vocal components of these tic disorders commonly include involuntary, repetitive sound productions, such as clicks, grunts, yelps, barks, sniffs, coughs, or words while the motor characteristics involve an assortment of various body movements, such as rapid eyeblinking, shoulder shrugging, head jerking, and facial twitching.

The clinical features of Tourette syndrome, as defined by the Diagnostic and Statistical Manual of Mental Disorders (DSM–IV[TM]) were profiled in Table 3–1. As is shown in Figure 5–3, the disorder first appears sometime during childhood, perhaps as early as age 2 but always by age 15. The symptoms, which include both multiple vocal and motor behaviors, persist for more than 1 year and vary in their intensity over time (e.g., exacerbation occurs with stress, conscious control suppresses movements for minutes to hours, overall behaviors wax and wane in frequency). Although not included in the current DSM criteria, several neurological and psycho-behavioral symptoms are commonly associated with TS, including attention deficit disorder, hyperactivity, learning disabilities, sleep disorders, enuresis, obsessive-compulsive behaviors, antisocial, impulsive, and sexually inappropriate behaviors, emotional lability, depressive reactions, and anxiety and phobic reactions (Cohen, Bruun, & Leckman, 1988).

Among the various assessments used to evaluate patients suspected of having TS is the neurological examination. According to Cohen, Leckman, and Shaywitz (1984), about half of the patients with Tourette syndrome present "soft" neurological signs and/or EEG abnormalities, suggesting disturbances in the body scheme and integration of motor control. They underscore the importance of baselining neurological performance in TS patients, prior to the initiation of drug therapy (usually haloperidol), since the effects of medications may cloud the neurological picture.

Apraxia

Although "pure" phonatory apraxia is rare, such cases do exist. More commonly, patients demonstrate a phonatory apraxia in combination with a coexisting speech and/or limb apraxia, or aphasia. Sometimes patients also exhibit a coexisting dysarthric component.

Both children and adults may present this type of motor speech disorder, which is characterized by an inability to produce volitional phonation. Despite the presence of normal laryngeal structures and normal laryngeal function on reflexive tasks such as coughing and swallowing, these patients exhibit laryngeal groping behaviors during their attempts to intentionally initiate voicing.

Other Dysarthias

Not infrequently, patients exhibiting early signs and symptoms of undiagnosed neurological diseases are referred to the voice care team with voice complaints. The vocal weakness, harsh-breathy quality, and monotone inflection associated with Parkinson's disease is one example. Other hyperkinetic and hypokinetic forms of dysarthria; cerebellar ataxia; and various progressive neurological diseases (e.g., ALS, MS) may also create problems with spasticity, flaccidity, coordination and/or control of the vocal tract structures that are first experienced as changes in speech and voice.

Referral to Psychiatry

Psychiatry, the medical discipline that deals with the study and treatment of mental disorders, is one of the most frequently needed, yet least commonly used, professions in many voice specialty clinics. Because patients present a range of psychological and behavioral dysfunctions that can affect the human voice and because the symptoms may masquerade as organic disorders or be associated with physical illnesses or conditions, differential diagnosis can often be difficult—without the knowledge and expertise of a skilled mental health professional.

Psychopathologies that are frequently encountered by the psychiatrist involved in liaison/consultative work with voice-disordered patients include:

anxiety disorders

conversion (somatoform) disorders

malingering

factitious disorders (Munchausen syndrome)

depressive (mood) disorders

personality disorders

These are charted in Figure 5–4.

Anxiety Disorders

Psychopathologies resulting in tensional symptoms due to overactivity in the autonomic and voluntary nervous systems comprise the greatest proportion of individuals suffering voice disorders of primarily psychogenic origin (Rammage, Nichol, & Morrison, 1987). Muscle tension is a common symptom associated with generalized anxiety disorders as well as somatoform disorders such as conversion disorder or hypochondriasis. Anxiety disorders are most commonly diagnosed in adults, but a detailed history may identify previously unrecognized manifestations that occurred during childhood or adolescence. In cases where an anxiety disorder is the primary etiology contributing to muscle hypertonicity affecting voice function, a combination of voice therapy and psychotherapy is indicated. The prognosis for voice rehabilitation may be dependent on the success of the psychological management.

Conversion Disorders

A conversion somatoform voice disorder may manifest itself as either aphonia or dysphonia. It is characterized by voice difficulty that suggests a neurological or other medical condition, but is actually related to unintentional abnormal muscle use. Although the symptoms may appear at any age, most patients presenting a conversion reaction are adolescents or young adults. The onset is typically sudden in nature and associated with psychological stressors (e.g., a traumatic event, stressful period, or troubling relationship), although some patients adamantly deny having any unusual life stresses or problems. They may also show suprising indifference about the voice disorder and assume a "la belle indifference" attitude about their vocal limitations (DSM–IV™).

Laryngeally, no physical evidence will be found to support an organic etiology. In keeping with DSM–IV™ descriptions, the clinical signs do not conform to known neurophysiological pathways or mechanisms. For example, the manifestations of conver-

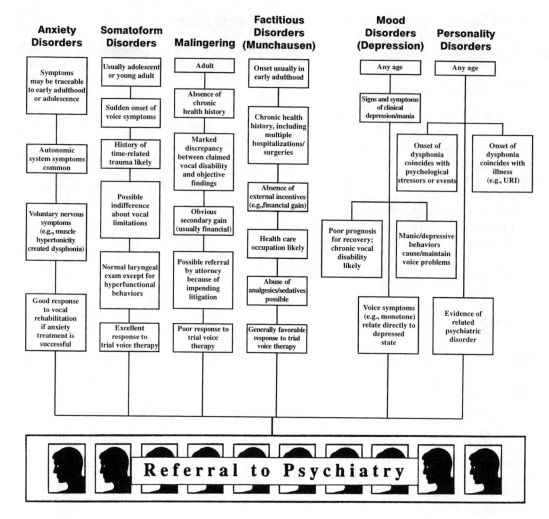

Figure 5–4. Referral to Psychiatry.

sion aphonia during speech are typically not consistent during reflexive vocalizations such as coughing or spontaneous laughter/crying. Muscle misuse behaviors are commonly demonstrated on laryngeal examination (e.g., anchored abductory positioning, vocal fold hyperadduction, anterior-posterior constriction, general compression of the supraglottic structures). In most cases, these individuals are quite responsive to trial voice therapy and usually have a good prognosis for recovery, unless the problem has been present for longer than 1 year, or significant predisposing/perpetuating personality traits or unresolved psychological

conflicts/gains exist (Nemiah, 1985; Rammage et al., 1987). More specific prognostic indicators for recovery from conversion symptoms include a stable and supportive psychosocial environment; ability to relate to the counsellor/physician/therapist; ability to be introspective, to feel and express emotions without developing incapacitating anxiety or depression, while maintaining psychological distance from consciously experienced emotion; symptoms that are fairly well circumscribed and related to identifiable environmental stressors; and associated psychological conflict that is primarily focused on genital, oedipal sexuality (Nemiah, 1985).

According to DSM–IV™, "Recurrence (of conversion symptoms) is common, occurring in one-fifth to one-quarter of individuals within a year." This suggests that all motivated patients should be referred for psychiatric consultation. However, the exact rate of recurrence, with and without psychiatric intervention, is not known.

Malingering

Unlike individuals with conversion disorders who are unconsciously producing voice symptoms, patients with disorders such as malingering and factitious disorders intentionally feign or grossly exaggerate their vocal disabilities. In the case of malingerers, there is no associated psychopathology, but typically some recognizable external incentive (e.g., financial gain, improved housing, disability insurance) motivating the behavior. In fact, some of these patients are actually sent to voice care professionals by attorneys in need of medical documentation to support a claim of vocal disability.

Generally, such patients report many more problems with their voices than would be expected given the objective, clinical findings; and they respond poorly to trial voice therapy, typically due to lack of cooperation and compliance. Malingering is suspect when the behaviors described are present in patients with antisocial personality disorder.

Because hypochondriacal patients with voice problems (individuals who tend to exaggerate their symptoms because of a fear or preoccupation with illness) and Munchausen patients (described below) can be mistaken for malingerers, consultation with a mental health professional can aid in differential diagnosis. Not surprisingly, few malingers welcome psychiatric referral!

Factitious Disorders: "Munchausen Syndrome"

In contrast to the malingerer, patients with factitious disorders feign, exaggerate, or intentionally produce symptoms of a disease or injury in order to assume the sick role, by seeking to undergo diagnostic tests, hospitalizations, or medical and surgical treatments. They typically present a chronic health history, involving multiple instances of hospitalization, and frequently have a past or current employment history as a nurse, physician, laboratory technician, ambulance driver, or other type of health care worker (Kaplan & Sadock, 1985).

When factitious disorders are found in middle-aged or older persons, onset of their initial symptoms can usually be traced back to early adulthood, followed by repeated episodes of factitious disorder or illness for which they may have received various types of medical and/or surgical interventions. Munchausen patients with predominantly physical manifestations tend to be abusers of sedatives and analgesics (DSM–IV™).

Trial voice therapy generally brings about temporary changes in voice (or breathing, in cases where the disorder manifests itself as Munchausen stridor) unless repeated surgeries or procedures have caused irreversible scarring or damage. Combined psychiatric counseling and symptomatic voice therapy are usually needed to treat these patients.

Mood Disorders

Varying degrees of depression and anxiety commonly accompany psychogenic voice disorders. As Aronson (1990) points out, depressive symptoms can either cause a voice disorder or develop in response to having voice problems. In either case, referral to a psychiatrist or other mental health professional may be necessary.

The relationship between depression, voice disorders, and the need for psychiatric referral has been shown in Figure 5–4. Three indicators for referral have been specified. They include instances in which:

1. The voice symptoms appear directly related to the patient's depressed state. These may involve musculoskeletal tension, affective voice signs (e.g., low-pitched, monotone, quiet voice), or other vocal abnormalities related to physical

or psychological symptoms of depressive states, such as reduced motivation, low energy, and fatigue.

2. The prognosis for voice recovery is poor. If patients are feeling depressed about their vocal limitations and the prognosis for voice recovery is poor, counseling may be helpful in helping them adjust to having a chronic disability. Examples include cancer patients who have lost all or part of their larynx, performers who are grieving over the loss of a career, substance abusers who are demonstrating maladaptive behaviors to their disabling condition, and many others.

3. Manic and/or depressive behaviors are serving to (at least in part) create or maintain voice problems. For some individuals, the presence of manic and/or depressive behaviors can be one of the primary sources of laryngeal abuse. The depressed patient, for example, may engage in frequent crying (vocal abuse), suffer from alcohol or other drug dependence, or exhibit altered speech and voice patterns secondary to associated anxiety (e.g., shallow, rapid breathing, accelerated rate of speech).

One such voice patient, later diagnosed with a manic/depressive illness, underwent voice therapy five times for the treatment of recurring, bilateral vocal nodules before she was finally referred to psychiatry. Once diagnosed and treated with medication, the behaviors that had been exacerbating her voice problems stabilized and no further recurrences have since been reported.

To assist practitioners in identifying depressed patients, some prominent clinical signs and symptoms of mood disorders have been listed in Table 5–3. Since patients may develop either a unipolar depression or a bipolar depression (manic-depressive illness), symptoms of both depression and mania have been included.

Personality Disorders

Certain patterns of behavior (e.g., perfectionism, impulsivity, inflexibility/rigidity, ad-

miration-seeking, compulsivity, behavioral eccentricities) may be indicative of personality disorders. The primary features of personality disorders are summarized as, "an enduring pattern of inner experience and behavior that deviates markedly from the expectations of the individual's culture and is manifested in at least two of the following areas: cognition, affectivity, interpersonal functioning, or impulse control" (DSM–IV™). Other criteria include application of these traits across a wide range of situations, and significant consequences on aspects of day-to-day functioning. The inflexible and maladaptive personality traits may predispose patients to chronic musculoskeletal tension, vocal abuse, and overuse (Aronson, 1990; Rammage et al., 1987). The psychosocial interview is a critical tool in uncovering evidence of narcissistic, obsessive-compulsive, histrionic, paranoid, schizoid, borderline, or other types of personality disorders (Shea, 1988).

Referral to Pulmonary Medicine

Pulmonary medicine, a subspecialty of internal medicine, deals with the study and treatment of lung disorders. Pulmonologists, the medical specialists who evaluate and treat respiratory problems, are routinely involved in the evaluation and management of pulmonary disorders, such as asthma, emphysema, bronchitis, pneumonia, cystic fibrosis, and occupational respiratory diseases. They also diagnose and manage pulmonary disturbances and complications related to: tuberculosis, AIDS, sleep apnea, lupus, scleroderma, sarcoidosis, rhematoid arthritis, kyphoscoliosis, spinal cord injuries, postpolio syndrome, amyotrophic lateral sclerosis, myasthenia gravis, Guillan-Barré syndrome, muscular dystrophy, vocal cord dysfunction, cancer, and a variety of other diseases and disorders. Tests of pulmonary function can assist in making a differential diagnosis, baselining pulmonary performance, identifying patients at risk for complications related to surgery and anesthesia, and establishing an efficacious treatment plan.

TABLE 5–3. Common signs and symptoms of mood disorders.

Depressive Features

Chronic depressed mood: pessimism, hopelessness, anxiety, despair

Reduced interest in work, hobbies, food, sex

Weight gain or loss, anorexia

Change in sleeping pattern: insomnia, hypersomnia

Change in psychomotor activity: restlessness/agitation, lethargy (hypomobility)

Lack of energy, fatigue

Feelings of guilt, worthlessness, self-doubt

Indecisiveness

Reduced attention, concentration

Suicidal thoughts

Slowed speech, lowered vocal pitch and intensity, monotone/monostress speech

Reduced interpersonal communication, social withdrawal

Manic Features

Heightened psychomotor activity: hyperactivity/restlessness/agitation

Heightened self-esteem

Grandiose ideas/activities: excessive or indiscrete investment/shopping/sexual activities

Reduced attention: distractibility

Inappropriate interpersonal behaviors/pragmatics

Pressed speech, elevated pitch and intensity, exaggerated inflection/stress patterns

Change in sleeping pattern: reduced need for sleep

Requests for pulmonary function evaluation are regularly received from professionals involved in voice care, because respiratory disorders often adversely influence voice production. Listed below are some pathologies that commonly require the collaborative services of a pulmonary specialist:

asthma

paradoxical motion of the vocal cords

progressive neurologic disease

interstitial lung disorders

These are charted in Figure 5–5.

Asthma

The current operational definition for asthma was first presented in 1992:

> Asthma is a chronic inflammatory disorder of the airways in which many cells play a role, including mast cells and eosinophils. In susceptible individuals this inflammation causes symptoms which are usually associated with widespread but variable airflow obstruction that is often reversible either spontaneously or with treatment, and causes an associated increase in airway responsiveness to a variety of stimuli. (International Consensus Report on the Diagnosis and Management of Asthma, 1992)

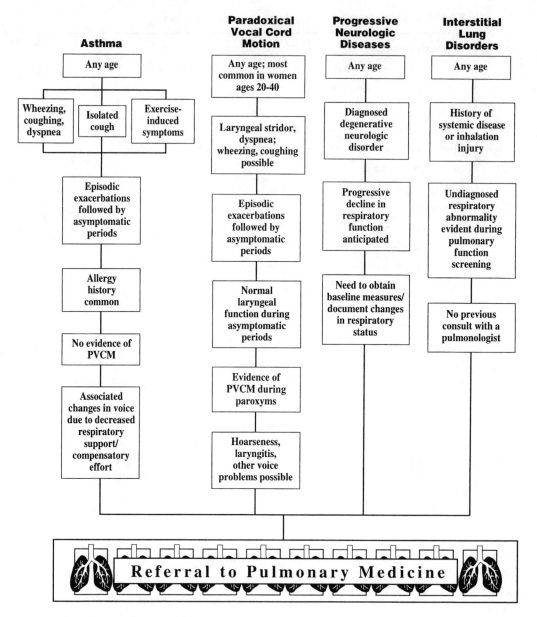

Figure 5–5. Referral to Pulmonary Medicine.

This physical condition, which can cause breathing difficulties in persons of all ages, affects approximately 8 million people in the United States and is considered to be the most prevalent obstructive airway disease (Sataloff, 1991). Historically, three cardinal symptoms have been associated with asthma: wheezing, coughing, and dyspnea. Although this triad still defines the most classic presentation of the disorder, recently asthma variants have emerged. One variant, for example, includes only an isolated cough, while another produces symptoms in response to exercise. In cases of exercise-induced asthma, symptoms such as wheezing, chest pain, and coughing generally develop either during or within 15 minutes of stopping exercise (Anderson, 1994).

Asthma "attacks" usually recur episodically, with acute exacerbations being interspersed with symptom-free periods. Although many asthma sufferers have a history of allergies, nonallergic asthma types also exist.

The relationship between asthma and the singing voice has been discussed by Sataloff (1991). He states that, in singers, even mild airway reactivity can interfere with performing by producing shortness of breath, vocal fatigue, decreased range, and impaired vocal control. Incorrect singing technique (e.g., jaw tension, tongue retraction, strap muscle hyperfunction) may also develop due to compensatory efforts. Although the symptoms may be difficult to recognize in milder or variant forms, pulmonary evaluation should be considered in suspected cases. Effective treatment options are available for both the professional and nonprofessional voice user.

Paradoxical Motion of the Vocal Cords

Vocal cord dysfunction (VCD), or paradoxical motion of the vocal cords (PMVC), is frequently misdiagnosed as "uncontrolled" asthma, or in some cases, vocal cord paralysis (Bless & Swift, 1993). Although these disorders share some common characteristics, their etiological and physiological bases are quite different.

In cases involving PMVC, there is adduction of the true vocal folds on inspiration with abduction on expiration. These asymptomatic (nonasthmatic) patients typically exhibit normal laryngeal structure and function on laryngoscopy, although some vocal cord mucous stranding may be present. Patients with an accompanying asthma frequently demonstrate coexisting voice problems, such as hoarseness, laryngitis, vocal nodules, or polyps (Martin, Blager, & Gay, 1987).

Patients with vocal cord dysfunction are predominately females between the ages of 20 and 40. Their medical history often includes previous treatments for upper airway obstruction, possibly involving emergency procedures such as tracheostomy or endotracheal intubation. As the result of long-term, high-dose steroid therapy, many have a Cushingoid appearance. In addition to reporting dyspnea, stridor, and coughing, patients may describe associated symptoms of hyperventilation and anxiety (e.g., dizziness, tingling in the fingers and toes, chest tightness). A history of stress or psychological problems is not uncommon.

Although laryngoscopy and videoendoscopy are routinely used to diagnose paradoxical vocal fold abnormalities, a complete assessment of pulmonary function (including tests of hyperreactivity and flow volume loops) is also indicated, in most cases, to identify any contributing allergic or asthmatic conditions and to assist in treatment planning.

Progressive Neurologic Disease

Patients diagnosed with degenerative disorders, such as amyotrophic lateral sclerosis (ALS), may need to undergo a series of pulmonary function studies in order to document the progressive changes in respiratory function that inevitably occur in response to the disease process. According to Miller (1987), the results of (repeated) pulmonary function testing can objectively plot the rate and course of respiratory decline in patients and offer practioners valuable prognostic information for use in patient counseling.

For the voice specialist who is concerned with maintaining functional communication, the results can provide guidance in planning needed augmentative and/or alternative communication systems. The use of speech amplifiers, electronic speech aids, electronic communication devices, and manual communication boards often proves to be facilitative to these patients, if and when reduced respiratory capacity prohibits normal voice production.

Interstitial Lung Disorders

Interstitial lung disorders (ILD) are "chronic, non-malignant, non-infectious diseases of the lower respiratory tract, characterized by inflammation and derangement of the alveolar walls" (Crystal, 1987). Examples of interstitial lung diseases include systemic disorders such as sarcoidosis, Sjogren's syndrome, systemic lupus erythematous, progressive systemic sclerosis, and rhematoid arthritis, as well as inhalation disorders that may develop following exposure to toxic substances.

Since the aforementioned disease processes can compromise breath support for speech (and, in some cases, also alter laryngeal structure and or function), speech pathologists routinely screen for deficiencies in respiration through the use of pulmonary function tests (e.g., spirometry), which are performed during comprehensive voice assessment.

Identification of a respiratory abnormality may indicate the need for referral to a specialist. Further pulmonary work-up is usually indicated in cases where the problem has gone undetected and/or the primary physician agrees that more extensive testing is necessary.

Referral to Speech Pathology

While medical speech pathologists often play a key role in assessing and diagnosing voice disorders, at times their involvement may be limited. For example, in smaller clinics, the caseload demands may not require the services of a full-time, on-site clinician. When this occurs, selected patients are generally referred by the physician to the speech pathologist for voice evaluation and/or behavioral treatment. The most common indications for voice therapy follow.

Five indications for referral have been indicated in Figure 5–6:

presurgical counseling

treatment of iatrogenic disorders

management of reversible, benign lesions/ conditions

management of "functional" disorders, without morphologic change

management of neurogenic disease/dysfunction

Presurgical Counseling

Essentially all voice patients scheduled to undergo laryngeal surgery benefit from presurgical consultation with a speech pathologist. The primary purpose of preoperative counseling is to inform patients about what to expect and do following their surgeries and to initiate any behavioral changes preoperatively that may interfere with recovery and/or success of the surgical procedure. In cases necessitating a total laryngectomy, patients are counseled regarding the postoperative anatomical changes that will affect both their voice and breathing. They are also provided with an overview of the various communication options that will be available to them as alaryngeal speakers.

When less invasive procedures are indicated, for example, in the treatment of laryngeal pathologies such as papilloma, mucous retention or demoid cysts, early glottic carcinomas, polyps, contact ulcer granulomas, or congenital laryngeal web, preoperative counseling addresses the vocal hygiene measures that will be used following phonosurgery, in order to reduce the risk of developing or maintaining inappropriate, compensatory behaviors and to minimize postoperative laryngeal trauma.

Treatment of Iatrogenic Disorders

Although all voice patients who have had medical or surgical management procedures do not require follow-up care with the speech pathologist, some do. For example, patients who demonstrate reduced mucosal wave and amplitude, secondary to postsurgical scarring, may benefit from a vocal excercise program emphasizing physiological therapy, such as vocal function exercises (Stemple, 1992).

Patients who have undergone laryngeal irradiation for glottic cancers often present voice abnormalities (e.g., decreased loudness, harshness, breathiness, low pitch) due to morphologic changes in the larynx (Morgan, Robinson, March, & Bradley, 1988). Such changes may include, but would not be lim-

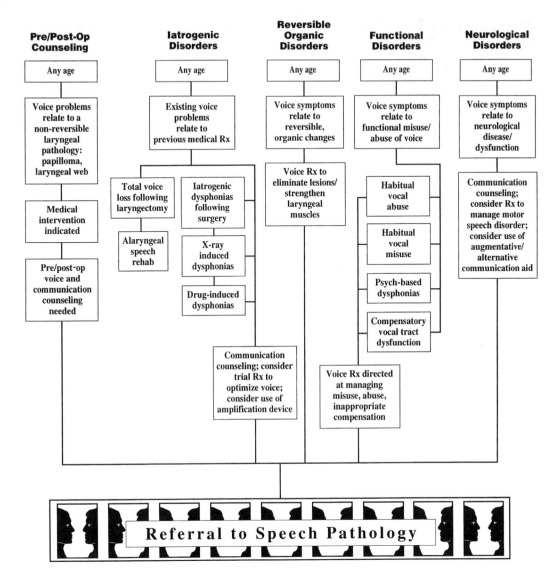

Figure 5–6. Referral to Speech Pathology.

ited to the following: laryngeal edema, fibrosis, and loss of mucous gland function (Chandler, 1979; Moench & Phillips, 1972; Morgan et al., 1988). These patients may also benefit from vocal function exercises, in addition to vocal hygiene counseling stressing the importance of hydration.

Among the other iatrogenic conditions that may be improved through voice therapy are postsurgical paresis or paralysis, vocal fold bowing secondary to long-term inhaler use, and overinjection of botulinum toxin. In each of these instances, careful documentation of session-to-session progress is important to justify the cost-effectiveness of voice therapy in such difficult to treat cases. Assuming therapy efficacy is well documented and despite the anatomic and physiologic limitations of a given patient, medical practitioners should not overlook potential contributions of trial voice therapy for selected iatrogenic voice problems.

Management of Reversible, Benign Lesions/Conditions

One of the most frequent therapy referrals made to speech pathology is for the treatment of reversible, benign lesions, such as vocal nodules and pseudocysts, or more specifically, the primary behavioral vocal abuses and muscle misuses that lead to development of these secondary lesions. Less common, but equally warranted, are therapy referrals made for the management of "hypofunctional" voice disorders (e.g., age-related vocal fold bowing or hypotonia) and counseling for precipitating conditions that produce laryngeal inflammation (gastroesophageal reflux).

Management of Behavioral Voice Disorders Without Morphologic Change

A wide range of behavior-based voice disorders, sometimes globally referred to as "functional" voice disorders, are routinely treated by the medical speech pathologist. These include muscle misuse voice problems due to poor vocal technique, adolescent transitional voice disorder ("falsetto"), psychological stress or conflict, hyper- and hypoadduction disorders, functional vocal fold bowing, glottal fry phonation, loudness disorders, pitch disorders, and chronic vocal abuse. This list also includes compensatory dysphonias related to primary speech, language, and/or hearing problems; for example, a child demonstrating both voice and fluency problems, who has underlying language/learning difficulties. In a case such as this, the treatment program of choice would incorporate combination therapy techniques, which would enhance all three aspects of the child's communication.

Management of Neurogenic Disease/Dysfunction

The clinical management of neurogenic communicative disorders usually involves at least some aspects of vocal rehabilitation. In the Parkinson patient, for example, therapy may emphasize increased vocal fold adduction and loudness, whereas in the ALS patient the management of velopharyngeal incompetence may be the primary clinical concern.

Patients with severe neurological deficits may require the use of alternative or augmentative communication systems. The speech pathologist will participate in the selection process of the appropriate unit and subsequently help the individual learn how to use the device effectively.

REFERENCES

Anderson, S. D. (1994). Diagnosis and management of exercise-induced asthma. In M. E. Gershwin & G. M. Halpern (Eds.), *Bronchial asthma: Principles of diagnosis and treatment* (3rd ed.). New Jersey: Humana Press.

Aronson, A. E. (1990). *Clinical voice disorders: An interdisciplinary approach* (3rd ed.). New York: Thieme Stratton.

Bless, D. M., & Swift, E. (1993, October). *Voice treatment of organic dysphonias.* Paper presented at Sixth Annual Pacific Voice Conference.

Chandler, J. R. (1979). Radiation fibrosis and necrosis of the larynx. *Annals of Otology, Rhinology and Laryngology, 88,* 509–514.

Cohen, D. J., Bruun, R. D., & Leckman, J. F. (1988). *Tourette's syndrome and tic disorders: Clinical understanding and treatment.* NY: John Wiley & Sons.

Cohen, D. J., Leckman, J. F., & Shaywitz, B. (1984). *A physician's guide to diagnosis and treatment of tourette syndrome.* Bayside, New York: Tourette Syndrome Association.

Colton, R. H., & Casper, J. K. (1990). *Understanding voice problems.* Baltimore: Williams & Wilkins.

Crystal, R. G. (1987). Interstitial lung disorders. In E. Braunwald, K. Isselbacher, R. Petersdorf, J. Wilson, J. Martin, & A. Fauci (Eds.), *Harrison's principles of internal medicine* (11th ed.). New York: McGraw-Hill.

Damste, P. H. (1964). Virilization of the voice due to anabolic steroids. *Folia Phoniatrica, 16,* 10–18.

Damste, P. H. (1967). Voice change in adult women caused by virilizing agents. *Journal of Speech and Hearing Disorders, 32,* 126–132.

Darley, F. L., Aronson, A. E., & Brown, J. R. (1975). *Motor speech disorders.* Philadelphia: W. B. Saunders.

Diagnostic and statistical manual of mental disorders (4th ed.) (DSM–IV™) (1994). Washington, DC: American Psychiatric Association.

Fried, M. P. (1988). *The larynx: A multidisciplinary approach.* Boston: Little, Brown.

International consensus report on the diagnosis and management of asthma. (1992). *Allergy, 47* (Suppl. 13).

Kaplan, H. I., & Sadock, B. J. (1985). *Comprehensive textbook of psychiatry IV.* Baltimore: Williams & Wilkins.

Koller, W. C. (1990). Evaluation of tremor disorders. *Hospital Practice* (Office Ed.), 25(5A), 23, 26–27, 30–31.

Martin, R. J., Blager, F. B., & Gay, M. I. (1987). Paradoxical vocal fold motion in presumed asthmatics. *Seminars in Respiratory Medicine, 8*(4), 332–337.

Miller, A. (1987). *Pulmonary function tests: A guide for the student and house officer.* Orlando, FL: Grune & Stratton.

Moench, M., & Phillips, R. (1972). Carcinoma of the nasopharynx. Review of 146 patients with emphasis on radiation dose and time factors. *American Journal of Surgery, 124*(4), 515–518.

Morgan, D. A., Robinson, H. F., Marsh, L., & Bradley, P. J. (1988). Vocal quality 10 years after radiotherapy for early glottic cancer. *Clinical Radiology, 39*(3), 295–296.

Nemiah, J. C. (1985). Somatoform disorders. In H. I. Kaplan & B. J. Sadock (Eds.), *Comprehensive textbook of psychiatry IV.* Baltimore: Williams & Wilkins.

Rammage, L. A., Nichol, H., & Morrison, M. D. (1987). The psychopathology of voice disorders. *Human Communication Canada, 11,* 21–25.

Sataloff, R. T. (1991). *Professional voice: The science and art of clinical care.* New York: Raven Press.

Schwab, J. J., Clemons, R. S., Valder, M. J., & Raulerson, J. D. (1966). Medical patients' reaction to referring physicians after psychiatric consultation. *Journal of the American Medical Association, 195,* 1120–1122.

Shea, S. C. (1988). *Psychiatric interviewing—The art of understanding.* Philadelphia: W. B. Saunders.

Stemple, J. C. (1992). *Voice therapy—Clinical studies.* St. Louis: Mosby-Year Book.

Tyler, H. R. (1988). Neurologic disorders. In M. P. Fried (Ed.), *The larynx: A multidisciplinary approach.* Boston: Little, Brown.

Woodson, G. E., Zwirmer, P., Murry, T., & Swenson, M. P. (1992). Functional assessment of patients with spasmodic dysphonia. *Journal of Voice, 6*(4), 338–343.

Yorkston, K. M., Beukelman, D. R., & Bell, K. R. (1988). *Clinical management of dysarthric speakers.* Boston: College-Hill Press.

CHAPTER

PLANNING AND MONITORING VOICE TREATMENTS

atients seeking treatment may have a variety of conditions that arise from a variety of etiologies. Each condition challenges the voice care team to understand the underlying nature of a patient's symptoms and to plan treatments that target those aspects of the problem that can be modified.

Certain conditions leading to laryngeal dysfunction require primary medical and/ or surgical treatments. Others are best addressed through behavioral therapy. In many cases, optimal results are reached with a combined treatment approach where medical/surgical interventions and behavioral therapy complement each other. Patients' progress can be determined most accurately when voice care professionals understand the optimal treatment combination, and the limitations of therapy in modifying certain conditions.

CURRENT TRENDS IN TREATMENT

Medical Treatments

Common conditions that bring patients to the voice care team for medical or surgical treatments include vocal fold paralysis, spasmodic dysphonia, benign laryngeal lesions, and laryngeal cancer.

Vocal Fold Paralysis

Under the otolaryngologists' purview, the paralyzed vocal fold might be injected with fillers such as Gelfoam, Teflon, or autogenous fat. Thyroplasty and reinnervation are also common surgical procedures used to improve vocal fold approximation.

Gelfoam, a temporary injectable substance that persists 4 to 12 weeks, continues to be used selectively in patients during the period of spontaneous recovery or to determine the probable outcome of permanent vocal fold augmentation.

Teflon, an alloplastics filler, has received the most widespread acceptance over the past 25 years as a permanent injectable substance. Benninger and Schwimmer (1995), and Tucker (1988) advocate the use of Teflon to achieve vocal fold medialization. Tucker proclaims that, performed properly, "This approach is inexpensive, safe, and carries a high likelihood of significant improvement in voice." However, the problems with Teflon—improper placement, migration, and vocal fold stiffness—have compelled practitioners to look for alternative injectable materials.

Bioimplants such as bovine collagen and autogenous fat have provided viable alternatives to Teflon since these materials not only augment the mass of the vocal fold but may also be incorporated into the tissue structure over time. In the case of soluble (bovine) collagen, the injected collagen is thought to be replaced with natural collagen in the lamina propria. Bless, Ford, and Loftus (1992), Ford (1991), and Ford and Bless (1986) have reviewed their experiences with collagen in treating unilateral recurrent paralysis, vocal fold bowing and atrophy (presbylaryngis), and scarring secondary to surgical trauma. Their findings support the use of collagen in cases requiring medialization when there is not a high degree of glottic insufficiency, and in cases involving laryngeal scarring.

Autogenous fat cells injected deep into the thyroaytenoid and vocalis muscle can develop their own blood supply if they survive the trauma of transplantation. This technique, first applied to phonosurgery in 1987 by Brandenburg, has been used successfully to augment and medialize the paralyzed vocal fold (Brandenburg, Kirkham, & Koschkee, 1992; Brandenburg, Unger, & Koschkee, 1996).

Laryngoplastic phonosurgery is an alternative method for achieving vocal fold medialization. Koufman (1986) and others have reported on the successful use of thyroplasty-Type I in patients with vocal fold paralyses. The procedure, introduced by Isshiki in 1975, involves use of a silastic implant that is inserted between the thyroid cartilage and inner perichondrium to medialize the paralyzed vocal fold. A combination procedure, thyroplasty and arytenoid adduction, may be indicated in patients with a persistent posterior chink (Koufman, 1988).

Finally, surgical reinnvervation, using either a neuromuscular pedicle transfer or a recurrent laryngeal nerve suture anastomosis, has been applied in selected cases of vocal fold paralysis. Tucker (1977), Takenouchi and Matsu (1971), and Crumley (1991) have reported on their experiences in restoring innervation to paralyzed muscles using this technique.

Patients who experience difficulty adjusting to their surgically altered voices following any vocal fold approximating procedure may benefit from postsurgical voice therapy. In these cases, probe therapy is used to determine which techniques minimize inappropriate compensatory adjustments, and maximize vocal quality, stability, and power under the new phonatory conditions.

Spasmodic Dysphonias

Spasmodic dysphonias (SD) are now often treated with injection of botulinum toxin to produce a temporary paresis in the vocal folds. Other treatments for spasmodic dysphonias include nerve resection, thyroplasty, and behavioral therapy.

Ludlow (1990); Ludlow, Naunton, Fujita, and Sedory (1990); Ludlow, Naunton, Terada, and Anderson (1991); and Ludlow, Bagley, Yin, and Koda (1992) have reported on the treatment effects of botulinum toxin at the National Institutes of Health (NIH). Other investigators, including Blitzer and Brin (1992) and Ford, Bless, and Patel (1992), have also studied its effects. In general, these investigations have demonstrated that injections of botulinum toxin into the muscles of the larynx can produce a temporary paralysis or paresis (generally lasting from 3 to 6 months) that alleviates muscle spasms and improves voice for many patients. Some patients and clinicians suspect that the duration of the drug's effect is increased by supplementing the injections with a voice therapy program that teaches patients how to reduce laryngeal resistance during phonation. Ludlow (1995) recommends that a maximum trial period of six voice therapy sessions be employed to determine if a combination treatment is beneficial for a particular patient.

Some laryngologists prefer to treat laryngeal dystonias with phonosurgery. Dedo, the originator of recurrent laryngeal nerve section (1976), continues to advocate this treatment approach, using repeated surgery and/or laser thinning of the vocal fold in cases of recurrence of the SD symptoms (Dedo & Behlau, 1991; Dedo & Izdebski, 1983). In contrast to Dedo's traditional surgical approach, Isshiki (1989) uses laryngeal framework surgeries (thyroplasty Type II or Type III) and Tucker (1992) describes a combination procedure that incorporates laryngeal nerve section and thyroplasty.

Benign Laryngeal Lesions

Patients may require medical and/or surgical treatment for a variety of benign lesions that are either congenital or acquired. Among the conditions most commonly treated with primary medical and/or surgical approaches are:

contact ulcers/granulomas, typically treated primarily with antireflux measures;

congenital sulcus (sulci) vocalis, typically treated with phonosurgical techniques to free mucosal edges of the vocal folds and/ or medialize the vocal folds with an injectable substance;

cysts (epidermoid or mucous retention type), usually surgically removed, and in some cases of epidermoid cyst, followed by phono-surgical techniques for residual sulcus vocalis;

vocal fold polyps/polypoid degeneration, usually treated with a combination of behavioral (e.g., reduce health abuses such as smoking; reduce vocal abuses/misuses); medical (e.g., antireflux measures); and sometimes phonosurgical approaches;

papillomatosis, treated primarily with surgical ablation (often multiple procedures over time).

For further details on surgical interventions, the reader is referred to excellent texts on this topic (e.g., Ford & Bless, 1991; Isshiki, 1989; Rubin, Sataloff, Korovin, & Gould, 1995).

The medical and/or surgical interventions are often supplemented with pre- and post-operative counseling and behavioral voice therapy. In most cases where surgery is the primary treatment, the laryngologist and speech pathologist work as a management team to ensure that patients understand the dynamic relationship between vocal health, organic disease, and muscle use/misuse, and to help them maximize the benefits of surgical treatments by minimizing vocal abuses and compensatory muscle misuses, and observing the prescribed instructions for postoperative recovery. Appendix 6–1 offers some suggestions for postoperative care. Variations in post-op protocols reflect differences in practices and philosophies from one clinic to the next, for example, considerable controversy still exists regarding how long, if at all, patients should maintain silence following surgery.

Laryngeal Cancers

Head and neck cancer surgeries often involve the vocal system. Patients may be left with a variety of iatrogenic conditions following those ablative surgeries.

Some patients with laryngeal cancer are candidates for conservation surgeries such as laser cordectomy or subtotal laryngectomy procedures. Others may benefit from radiation therapy. Current computer technology and the latest x-ray and electron-generating machines (e.g., linear accelerators) now allow oncologists to effectively destroy cancer cells while better protecting normal cells from the toxic effects of radiation.

In cases requiring a complete laryngectomy, voice restoration may be facilitated with innovative surgical techniques such as the tracheoesophageal puncture (TEP) developed by Singer and Blom (1980). The TEP voice restoration procedure allows air to pass through a surgically created fistula kept open by a prosthetic device, enabling the laryngectomized patient to speak with a greater and more powerful air supply than is available to the traditional esophageal speaker (Blom, 1995; Robbins, Fisher, Blom, & Singer, 1984).

Another surgical technique, the neoglottis, has restored voice to alaryngeal speakers without the aid of a prosthesis. This reconstructive surgery utilizes upper tracheal cartilage to create a new source of vibration in the esophagus (Brandenburg, 1980; Brandenburg, Cragle, & Rammage, 1991).

Behavioral Treatments

Although the effects of successful voice therapy will be evident to health care professionals involved in a patient's follow-up management, few specialists outside the field of speech pathology are familiar with the processes involved in behavioral therapy for voice disorders. All too commonly, patients are referred to speech pathology for voice therapy by practitioners who have little appreciation of the scope and complexities of behavioral treatment programs. This is most common among practitioners who do not have access to well-equipped vocal function laboratories and interdisciplinary voice care teams. Speech pathologists working outside this type of facility may also have limited knowledge and access to instrumental methods used routinely by specialized clinicians in planning and monitoring contemporary voice thera-

py programs targeting specific disorder patterns. Lack of knowledge about current approaches in medical and behavioral management may lead clinicians to engage in therapy activities that are ineffective or to fail to refer clients in need of specialized care to the appropriate facilities.

Practitioners across disciplines need to acquire a better understanding of the current trends in voice therapy to clarify when referral is indicated and to establish mutual realistic expectations of therapy outcomes.

Current approaches to behavioral management center around identification of the underlying physiological changes needed to improve perceptual characteristics of the voice and/or an individual's technical use of the vocal system. Treatment programs that are carefully designed to target specific changes in vocal physiology permit an integration of theoretical models into clinical practice, allow clinicians to apply objective pre-, intra-, and post-therapy comparisons to evaluate progress, and lend themselves to the rigors of scientific testing through treatment efficacy studies.

Figure 6–1 illustrates the basic components of therapeutic work, viewed from a physiologically based orientation. This schema combines three critical elements that revolve around a central force: physiological measurements. The resulting system involves documentation of physiological function, either before or after each of the following steps:

► Identifying the desired physiological change(s) to be made through voice therapy,
► Administering stimulability probes to determine prognosis, and the most effective therapeutic procedures for accomplishing change, and
► Implementing selected procedures.

Identifying Areas in Need of Change

The voice assessment results identify areas in need of behavioral change. Both individual patient profiles, generated from observational and instrumental assessment, and the working diagnosis assist clinicians in selecting appropriate treatment objectives.

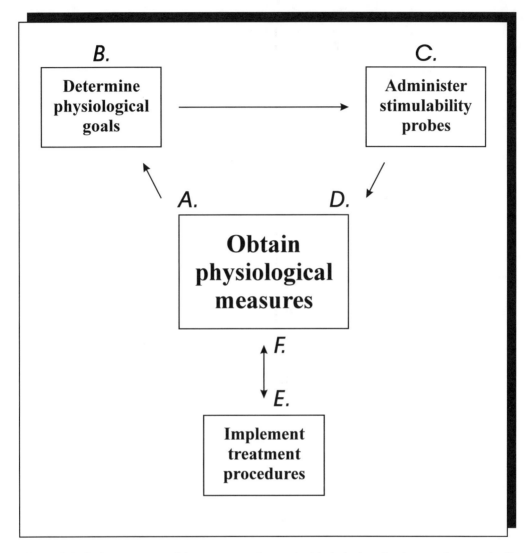

Figure 6–1. Basic components of therapy process, from a physiological orientation (see text for more detail).

An individual patient profile (Figure 6–2) can easily identify specific vocal function measures that fall outside the "normal" range of functioning. For some patients (e.g., closed head-injury cases), all objective test measures may fall well outside of the normal range. It might be unrealistic to expect these patients to make more than minimal improvements in one or two targeted areas due to significant anatomic and physiological limitations. In contrast, individuals with muscle misuse voice disorders may be capable of making a number of physiolo-

gical changes that will drastically affect their vocal function and quality. In this population, it is not unusual for clusters of behaviors to change simultaneously in response to modifications in vocal technique.

In treating patients who use their voices occupationally or professionally, diagnostic profiles that show all parameters falling within or above the "normal" range of production are sometimes generated. Nonetheless, given the nature of their vocal demands, these patients find that their vocal outputs do not meet the standards necessary for

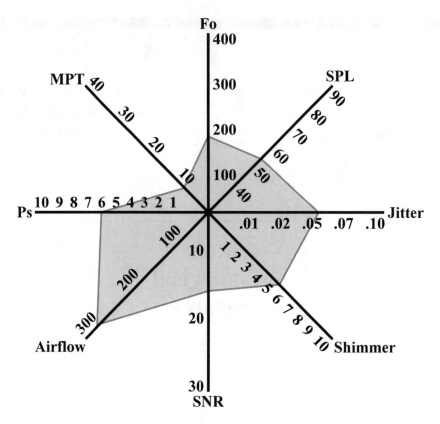

Figure 6–2. Individual Patient Profile, including a "normal" range (shaded area) for comparison against patient values. (Reproduced with permission from Bless, 1990.)

performing, and/or they experience vocal fatigue or discomfort in association with their occupational or professional voice use. In these cases, the primary therapy objectives may target refinements in muscle use and vocal technique. Minimizing suprahyoid muscle tension or irregularities in vocal fold movements or altering the singer's formant spectrographically are examples of clinical objectives that might be targeted in therapy to accommodate the extraordinary vocal demands required of the vocal performer.

The etiological bases of the voice problem can also offer guidance in planning behavioral intervention. Outlined in Table 6–1 are 17 physiological measures commonly targeted for change in therapy. This list identifies specific acoustic, aerodynamic, and kinematic variables frequently in need of modification for selected voice disorders.

Although individual variations from these clinical patterns will undoubtedly occur, these "classic" characteristics, which have been commonly associated with the identified conditions, can provide some clinical guidance in establishing target behaviors.

For example, hypophonic speakers with Parkinson's disease (col. 1 in Table 6–1) generally benefit from vocal exercises that (3) increase fundamental frequency range, (4) raise habitual intensity, (6) expand vocal intensity range (at the upper end of the intensity scale), (9) elevate subglottal pressure, (11) increase phonatory volume, (12) increase phonatory stability, (13) improve glottic closure, and (17) increase amplitude of vibration. Knowledge of these related physiological areas of deficit, typical of Parkinson's disease, can help clinicians establish the treatment objectives that may become the focus of behavioral voice therapy.

TABLE 6–1. Physiological measures targeted in the treatment of selected voice disorders.

MEASURES	PD	VN	VFS	RLN	HADD	MF	MTD	ADD SD
Increase f_0								
Decrease f_0			●			●		
Increase f_0 Range	●	●	●			●		
Increase SPL	●		●			●		
Decrease SPL								
Increase SPL Range	●		●	●		●		
Increase Airflow Rate								●
Decrease Airflow Rate				●			●	
Increase Pressure	●			●				
Decrease Pressure					●			●
Increase Air Volume	●							
Increase Phonatory Stability	●	●	●	●	●	●	●	●
Increase Glottic Closure	●	●	●	●		●	●	
Decrease Vocal Fold Hyperadduction		●			●			●
Decrease Supraglottic Constriction			●		●			●
Increase Mucosal Wave			●					
Increase Amplitude of Vibration		●	●	●	●	●		●

Pathology Code Legend:
PD = Parkinson's Disease
VN = Vocal Nodules
VFS = Vocal Fold Scarring
RLN = Recurrent Laryngeal Nerve Paralysis
HADD = Hyperadducting Dysphonia
MF = Mutational Falsetto
MTD = Muscle Tension Dysphonia
ADD SD = Adductor Spasmodic Dysphonia

The Contributions of Stimulability Testing

Once therapy objectives have been established, the clinician generally administers probe therapy to determine the effectiveness of specific behavioral procedures. Probe therapy or stimulability testing is a method for determining a patient's modifiability, using selected facilitating techniques. Probe batteries, a composite of several elicitation approaches, are often used to sample the differences among therapeutic procedures, particularly in special populations. Tables 6–2 and 6–3 present sample probe therapy batteries which were designed for use with spasmodic dysphonia and paralysis patients, respectively.

The spasmodic dysphonia battery (Table 6–2) assesses the patient's ability to produce different vowels (e.g., the low backed vowel /ɑ/, the high fronted vowel /i/, and the

TABLE 6–2. Stimulability testing for spasmodic dysphonia.

PROBE:		EFFECTIVENESS	CONSISTENCY		COMMENTS
			#+/#trials	%+	
Different vowels:	/ɑ/	+ / -	/	%	
	/i/	+ / -	/	%	
	/u/	+ / -	/	%	
Singing:	/ɑ/	+ / -	/	%	
	falsetto	+ / -	/	%	
	glissando	+ / -	/	%	
Humming:	/m/extended	+ / -	/	%	
Mandibular movements:	/ɑnɑ/*	+ / -	/	%	
	/ɑvɑ/*	+ / -	/	%	
Coordinated Voice Onset:	/hm/	+ / -	/	%	
	/m hm/	+ / -	/	%	
	/hɑ/	+ / -	/	%	
Inspiratory phonation:	/i/extended	+ / -	/	%	
	counting	+ / -	/	%	
Relaxation:	Yawn-Sigh	+ / -	/	%	
	Head-Shake	+ / -	/	%	
Reduced glottal attack:	/h/onset	+ / -	/	%	
Higher flow:	breathy voice	+ / -	/	%	
Altered loudness:	"Hey!"	+ / -	/	%	
	/ɑ/extended	+ / -	/	%	
	counting	+ / -	/	%	
Other (specify):		+ / -	/	%	

*repeated continuously at typical speech rate

rounded backed vowel /u/), compares sung versus spoken productions, and determines the effects of loudness, mandibular motion, nasality, and general relaxation on voice production. This probe battery also examines inspiratory speech, falsetto phonation, and various types of voice onsets.

Administration of the probe battery involves two procedures: elicitation of treatment probes and analysis of the samples to determine if desired psychoacoustic and/or physiological changes result. Vocal tasks that are performed well with consistency become the starting point in therapy and

TABLE 6–3. Stimulability testing for vocal fold paralysis.

TREATMENT PROBE:	IMPROVED QUALITY	SPL CHANGE (dB SPL	INCREASED CLOSURE	FLOW (ml/sec)	DECREASED HYPERFUNCTION
Increase closure:					
a. Pushing / pulling					
1. arm pump	+ / –		+ / –		+ / –
2. pulling	+ / –		+ / –		+ / –
3. pushing	+ / –		+ / –		+ / –
b. Primitive closure					
1. coughing	+ / –		+ / –		+ / –
2. laughing	+ / –		+ / –		+ / –
Decrease 2⁰ misuse					
a. Glottal attack					
1. start with /s/	+ / –		+ / –		+ / –
2. start with /h/	+ / –		+ / –		+ / –
3. start with /m/	+ / –		+ / –		+ / –
b. Relaxation					
1. sigh	+ / –		+ / –		+ / –
2. yawn-sigh	+ / –		+ / –		+ / –
Decrease abuses:					
a. Abuses identified	+ / –		+ / –		+ / –
Modify Pitch:					
a. Three tone scales					
1. higher pitch	+ / –		+ / –		+ / –
2. lower pitch	+ / –		+ / –		+ / –
Increase support:					
a. Increase lung volume	+ / –		+ / –		+ / –
b. Increase abdominal support	+ / –		+ / –		+ / –

Patient is responsive to probe(s); initiate therapy: Y   N
Patient needs vocal hygiene program: Y   N
Comments:

Source: Adapted from National Center for Voice and Speech (1991).

sometimes lead to specific treatment programs such as the CVO-coordinated voice onset and extension technique (Morrison & Rammage, 1994; Rammage, 1996) or the voice on inhalation technique (Shulman, 1993).

This scoring system uses +/− scores, consistency scores (e.g., number of positive responses in a trial of five attempts), and ob-servational commentary for recording patient responsiveness to individual treatment probes. The total time required to complete the protocol and score a patient's responses usually ranges from 10 to 20 minutes. The results of SD probe testing can aid clinicians in planning therapy programs and predicting prognosis for patients who have a spasmodic dysphonia, but who:

▶ Do not desire medical management,
▶ Wish to undergo a trial of voice therapy prior to deciding about medical intervention,
▶ Are too young to be considered for botulinum injection or laryngeal surgeries,
▶ Appear to have a primary psychogenic etiology for the disorder,
▶ Exhibit only mild SD symptoms, or,
▶ Have associated behaviors or problems that are not alleviated through medical management alone.

The second sample probe protocol (Table 6-3) was designed for stimulability testing in patients with unilateral vocal fold paralysis. The methodology is similar to the SD probe. The clinician uses +/− scoring and specific instrumental measures to make comparisons with baseline measures for laryngeal quality, vocal intensity, degree of glottic closure, mean airflow rate, and hyperfunctional behaviors. Procedurally, a variety of tasks are sampled to:

▶ Increase glottic closure,
▶ Decrease secondary hyperadducting muscle misuse ("hyperfunction"),
▶ Identify vocally abusive behaviors,
▶ Modify habitual pitch, and
▶ Improve respiratory support.

The total length of time typically required to administer this probe battery is 20 to 30 minutes. In essence, diagnostic probes are treatment trajectories that lead to specific therapeutic methodologies.

Unlike traditional speech stimulability testing, which emphasizes the importance of progressing from single sound or syllable productions to longer and more complex sequences, voice probes explore a wide range of productions, from isolated vowels to conversational speech. If several techniques prove equally effective, the technique representing the highest level of production is generally selected as the starting point of therapy, to minimize the duration of treatment and maximize motivation. For example, in a patient with a hyperadducting

muscle misuse dysphonia (with tight approximation of the arytenoids, lateral compression of the true vocal folds, long closed phase to the vibratory cycle, and possible lateral and/or A-P compression of supraglottic structures), three treatment approaches—the yawn-sigh technique (Boone & McFarlane, 1988), the aspirate initiation approach (Colton & Casper, 1990), and the confidential voice (Colton & Casper, 1990)—may all bring about the same desired physiological and psychoacoustic changes. In this instance, there would be several advantages to selecting the confidential voice as the treatment approach of choice, since this holistic technique usually allows patients to begin making modifications at the conversational level immediately. The other approaches require the patient to progress through a series of production levels before the techniques can be successfully applied to conversational speech.

On-line confirmation of each technique's effectiveness can be obtained with instrumental testing. For instance, in the case of the individual with a hyperadducting muscle misuse voice disorder, videostroboscopy, possibly complemented by electroglottography, inverse-filtered flow glottograms, or related measures could confirm that desired changes in glottic closure patterns had actually occurred. These could include reduced medial compression of the true vocal folds, less constriction of the false vocal folds and other supraglottic structures, and/or a reduced closed phase to the vibratory cycle. Other instrumental indicators that might be used to signify a reduction in laryngeal hyperadduction include increased mean airflow rate, reduced subglottal pressure, lowered mean fundamental frequency and/or a reduced habitual intensity level.

Implementing Selected Procedures

The basic emphasis on physiological processes should not minimize the importance of psychological aspects of voice disorders. Rather, the focus on physiology reflects our understanding of the underlying mechanisms of dysfunction, whether they are organic disease, psychosomatic illness, or a combination of these factors.

Psychosocial factors strongly influence clinicians in their decision-making with respect to diagnosis and implementation of individualized therapy programs. A patient's learning style (auditory vs. visual vs. kinesthetic), motivation, expectations (rapid vs. steady progress, partial vs. total recovery), cognitive level, lifestyle, and awareness of stress reactions are just some of the variables considered in planning a customized therapy program.

A wide range of therapeutic procedures have become available to clinicians involved in vocal rehabilitation. In addition to visual and biofeedback techniques, both traditional methods, such as vocal hygiene counseling and specific muscle relaxation therapies, and nontraditional methods, for example, whole-system approaches such as the Accent Method (Kotby, 1994) or the Stemple-Barnes-Briese Vocal Function Exercises (Stemple, 1993) are used in voice therapy to treat a wide range of voice disorders.

Prior to introducing any intervention program, the clinician must establish a performance baseline to allow for effective documentation of changes that occur as the result of therapy. A minimum of two baselines on all tasks has been recommended by

Bless (1991) to ensure reliability of performance. Two baseline measures can be obtained without delaying therapy when the first baseline is made during the initial diagnostic session and the second baseline is made at the beginning of the first therapy session. Because this protocol does not postpone the start of treatment, it does not raise issues regarding cost-effectiveness but does strengthen treatment efficacy.

Absolute stability is not a realistic expectation for human behavior. However, the question arises as to how much variability can be tolerated between baseline measures. Christensen (1977) has suggested that a stable baseline should fall within a 5% range. Certainly this is desirable and occurs approximately 90% of the time. However, in the remaining 10% of the cases, baseline instability may be demonstrated.

The presence of an unstable baseline can be due to variability in patient function, inconsistencies in examiner behaviors, or instrumental artifacts. If instrumental and examiner variability can be ruled out, the clinician should anticipate that further variability in the patient's behavior will occur during the course of treatment. Discovering why changes are demonstrated from day to day can facilitate therapy planning as the following case example demonstrates.

Patient 6-1.
Unstable Baseline/Patient Variability

This 18-year-old patient had sustained severe head injuries in an automobile accident two years earlier. Despite the severity of her injuries, she had recovered remarkably well, with the exception of a residually weak and breathy voice quality, related to recurrent laryngeal nerve paresis.

Initial evaluation of the patient had revealed conversational intensity level below norms: 60 dB; mean airflow rate above norms: 300cc/sec; and subglottal pressure below norms: 2.4 cm H_2O. Glottic closure was incomplete: a small longitudinal gap was present along the entire length of the membranous portion of the folds during phonation. These findings seemed to be consistent with the patient's history and reported concerns.

During her first treatment session, a second baseline was obtained to ensure test/retest reliability. Surprisingly, the patient demonstrated marked improvements in vocal function

(continued)

(continued)

measures. On the day of retesting and prior to intervention, she produced a conversational intensity level of 66 dB, a mean airflow rate of 230 cc/sec., and a subglottal air pressure of 4.2 cm H_2O. A videostroboscopic study revealed inconsistent glottic closure, with touch closure predominating during phonation produced at normal pitch and loudness.

Because of the variability demonstrated during the patient's first two clinic visits, she was asked to keep a 7-day voice diary (Figure 6–3) to explore the sources of variability (e.g., voice usage, fatigue, illnesses, and stress). Perusal of the diary revealed a tendency for improved voice to occur when the patient was well rested. On days when she reported being "totally exhausted," voice quality deteriorated appreciably.

Variability in performance is a clinical reality for some patients, especially those with neurological problems. For these individuals, erroneous judgments regarding pretreatment performance can sometimes occur if the type of clinical "detective" work described above is not undertaken. Furthermore, session-to-session variability may influence the patient's treatment schedule, since therapy schedules should accommodate the patient's communication needs and subsequent therapy objectives. In the case of Parkinson's patients, for instance, substantial alterations in behavior can be expected depending on the stage of their drug cycle. Ramig, Bonitati, and Winholtz (1994) advocate staggering the time of therapy sessions throughout the course of the day, to demonstrate to individuals with Parkinson's disease that they can make changes in loudness under varying conditions.

MONITORING THE COURSE OF CHANGE

Voice therapy, unlike many other types of speech rehabilitation, is generally short-term in nature (often not more than 12 weeks) and produces measurable results that can be monitored throughout the course of treatment. In most cases, measurable change will be seen within the first three therapy sessions. If not, a reexamination should be made of the therapeutic intervention to determine why the expected progress has not been made.

Three typical facets of behavioral modification offer guidelines in monitoring change: the patient, the methodology, and the clinician (Figure 6–4).

The Patient

Patient selection criteria form an important predictor of success in achieving behavioral changes. Just as patients are selected for surgical intervention on the basis of prognostic indicators for success (e.g., the etiology of the voice disorder, the presenting complaints and symptoms, and the likelihood for improvement following treatment), so should patients meet some basic criteria to become candidates for behavioral management. The schematic in Figure 6–5 provides guidance for clinicians referring patients for voice therapy.

An absence of other viable treatment options is not sufficient justification to recommend voice therapy, unless the patient needs counseling regarding communication difficulties and/or assistance in establishing an augmentative communication system (e.g., amplification).

When there is uncertainty about the possible benefits of behavioral management, referral for voice evaluation is always indicated and can even assist in creating realistic patient expectations about future progress.

"Bad timing" for behavioral intervention can be a saboteur of voice therapy. In some cases, treatment efforts that might be effective at a different point in time prove unsuc-

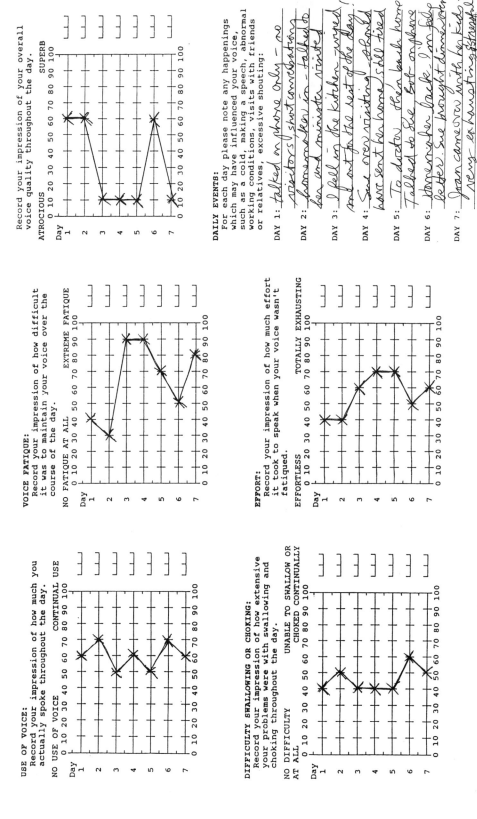

Figure 6–3. Daily voice diary for 1 week: the diary completed by Patient I reveals that fatigue is associated with vocal function. (Adapted with permission from National Center for Voice and Speech Quality of Voice 7-Day Diary, Version 7AI. University of Iowa; Denver Centre for the Performing Arts; University of Wisconsin-Madison; University of Utah.)

171

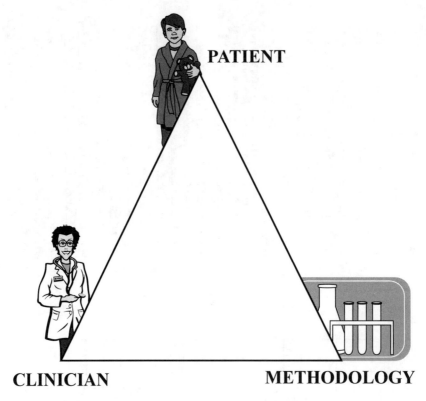

Figure 6–4. The Therapy Triad depicts three interactive areas of focus in behavioral therapy: all three points of focus need to be considered in monitoring changes during treatment.

cessful due a patient's inability to devote the required time and energy to his or her therapy program. Patients who are experiencing major life stresses or events (e.g., those caring for an ill spouse or suffering an episode of depression) may fall into this category. Certain major life changes and psychosocial events are considered to be stressful for most people (Table 2–6, Chapter 2).

Patients who have not yet made a commitment to giving up abusive habits (e.g., smoking, excessive drinking, cheerleading, talking in large groups without the use of amplification) may not be ready to accept their responsibility in the therapy process. Certainly, patients can be counseled and encouraged, as a part of therapy, regarding the many benefits of making change, but the patient's willingness and ability to comply with therapeutic advice is critical to successful intervention.

The Methodology

The development of an efficacious vocal rehabilitation program is the cornerstone of successful voice therapy. According to Karnell (1991), "As with medical and surgical treatments, the success of voice therapy largely depends on the selection of an appropriate treatment for the problem at hand" (p. 213).

To date, only a few well-designed therapy efficacy studies can guide the speech pathologist in behavioral program selection and development (e.g., Ramig, Bonitati, & Horii, 1991; Ramig, Bonitati, Lemke, & Horii, 1994; Ramig, Countryman, Thompson, & Horii, 1995). In light of the paucity of efficacy research, it is critical that individual effects of selected treatment approaches be carefully documented and systematically

DECISION-MAKING PROCESS FOR
VOICE ASSESSMENT AND MANAGEMENT

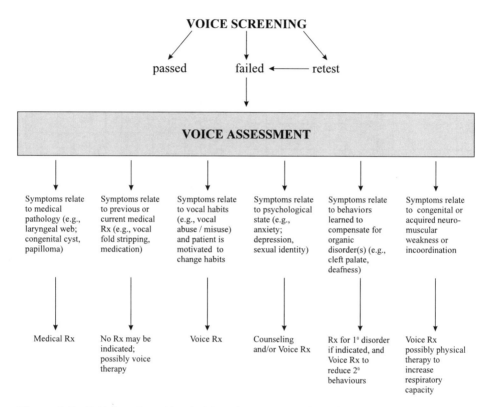

VOICE SCREENING

passed   failed ◄——— retest

VOICE ASSESSMENT

Symptoms relate to medical pathology (e.g., laryngeal web; congenital cyst, papilloma)	Symptoms relate to previous or current medical Rx (e.g., vocal fold stripping, medication)	Symptoms relate to vocal habits (e.g., vocal abuse / misuse) and patient is motivated to change habits	Symptoms relate to psychological state (e.g., anxiety; depression, sexual identity)	Symptoms relate to behaviors learned to compensate for organic disorder(s) (e.g., cleft palate, deafness)	Symptoms relate to congenital or acquired neuro-muscular weakness or incoordination
Medical Rx	No Rx may be indicated; possibly voice therapy	Voice Rx	Counseling and/or Voice Rx	Rx for 1° disorder if indicated, and Voice Rx to reduce 2° behaviours	Voice Rx possibly physical therapy to increase respiratory capacity

Figure 6–5. Guidelines for making decisions about patient referral for voice therapy.

studied to ensure that patients are progressing satisfactorily.

One system for monitoring physiological change—the Treatment Efficacy Response Form (TERF) (Figure 6–6) (Koschkee, 1991) —was specifically designed for the continued monitoring of selected aerodynamic and acoustic measures. Although this clinical tool was originally developed to focus on physiological changes resulting from voice therapy, its usefulness and clinical applicability extend beyond behavioral management to other types of intervention, such as surgical, pharmacological, and radiation therapy treatments. The TERF incorporates three important features for documenting vocal function changes:

► establishment of of a stable baseline prior to therapeutic intervention,
► a session-by-session recording of "key" vocal function measures, and
► a graphic display of progress.

One, two, or three baseline measures may be recorded on the TERF before treatment is initiated. A minimum of two is required for efficacious therapy planning. Although no specific vocal task has been identified, it is recommended that all measurements be made during production of the sustained vowel /a/ since normative values are most accessible for this vowel sound. If other tasks are selected for baselining, then the same tasks must be consistently repeated

TREATMENT EFFICACY RESPONSE FORM

PATIENT: _____

DIAGNOSIS: _____

POST BASELINE TREATMENT: _____

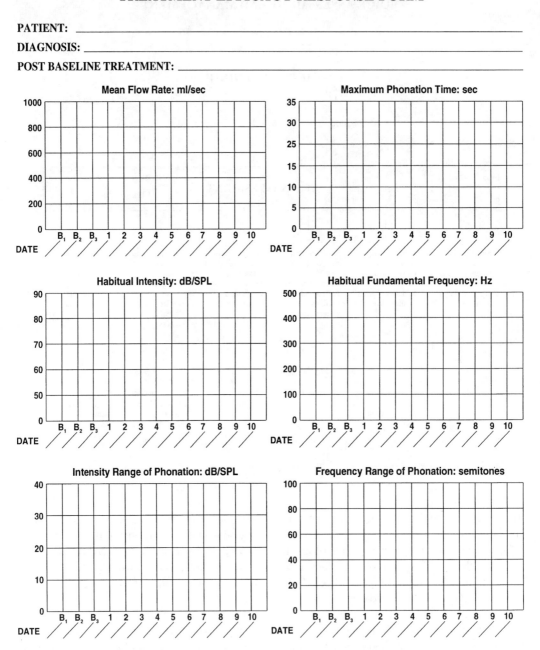

Figure 6–6. Treatment Efficacy Response Form (TERF). (Reprinted from "Treatment Response Form" by D. L. Koschke, 1991. Presented at ASHA Scientific Advances Conference, Madison, WI, with permission.)

during subsequent testing, and appropriate norms must be used for accurate data interpretation.

The use of charting systems such as the TERF offers several advantages. First, by continuously monitoring behaviors over time, clinicians can objectively judge the effectiveness of treatment programs. Second, by viewing their progress charts, patients can be encouraged to continue effecting behavioral changes (e.g., decreasing vocal abuse, practicing newly acquired behaviors). Third, when used in conjunction with supplemental overlays showing the typical range of performance for the patient's particular normative subgroup (e.g., adult male, adult female, 8–10 year-old child), treatment efficacy response forms can assist in counseling patients about their voice problems and aid in clarifying therapy objectives (Figure 6–7).

Typical Values for Adult Males

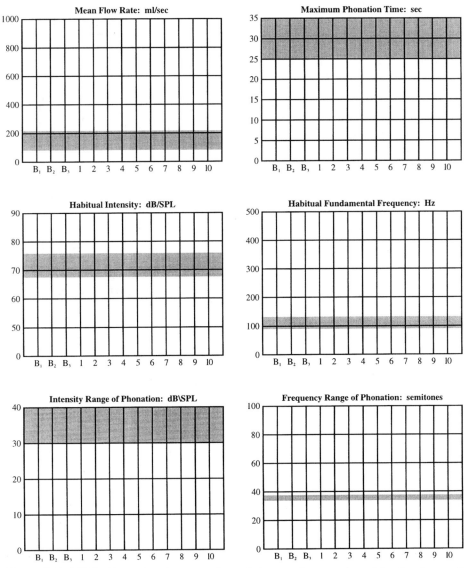

Figure 6–7. TERF with overlays demonstrating typical ranges for normal vocal function for specific age/sex populations. **A.** Typical vocal function values for adult males. **B.** Typical vocal function values for adult females. **C.** Typical vocal function values for children, aged 8–10. *(continued)*

Figure 6–7. *(continued)*

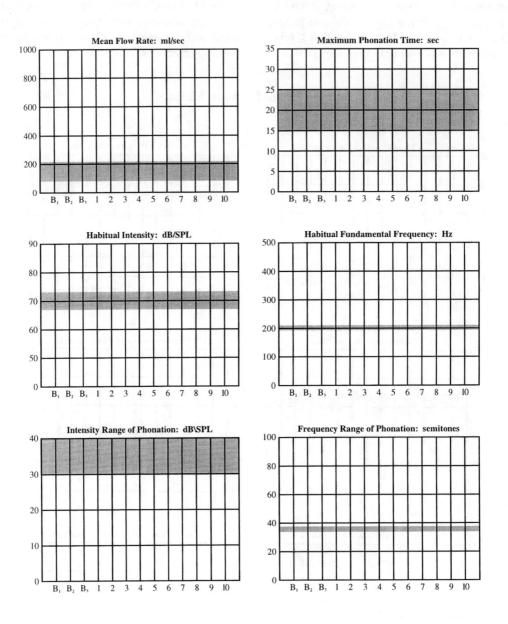

Typical Values for Adult Females

Other methodological issues commonly confronted by the clinician are determining the frequency of therapy sessions and the inclusion of home programming strategies in the framework of the treatment hierarchy. Although the frequency of therapy sessions should be based primarily on program-matic needs, practical considerations (e.g., traveling a distance to receive therapy, scheduling around work and other commitments) inevitably influence this clinical decision. Some treatment programs lend themselves to a therapy schedule that is convenient for the patient (e.g., once a week therapy for a

Typical Values for Children
(8-10 years)

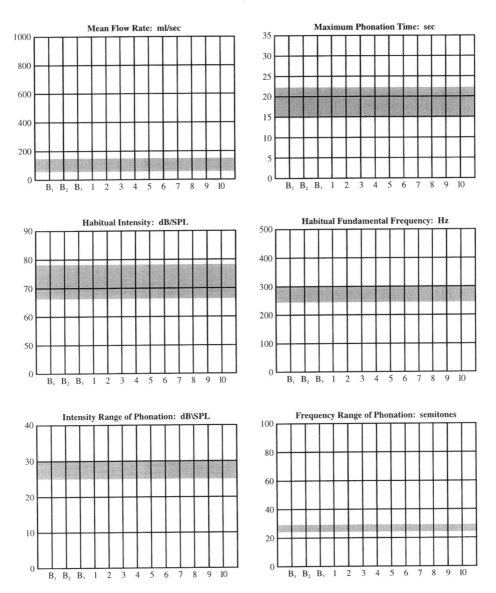

vocal abuse reduction program); other therapy techniques require more intensive voice therapy. Examples of intensive vocal rehabilitation programs that involve three or more treatment sessions per week include the Lee Silverman Voice Treatment for Parkinson's disease and the Accent Method of Voice Therapy.

In cases where intensive practice is needed but the patient is unable to attend therapy in the medical setting, creative problem-solving on the part of the clinician can often help to fill the therapeutic void. Among the possible solutions to the scheduling dilemma are telephone therapy, engaging speech aides or other nonprofessional or semi-professional personnel, intensive voice therapy implemented over a 1- to 2-week period, and programmed home practice.

Adjunct telephone therapy can successfully augment in-clinic therapy for some individuals. Geriatric patients in nursing home settings or other patients for whom travel requirements prohibit regular clinic visits may be candidates for this type of supplemental programming. Structured therapy programs, such as the Lee Silverman Treatment, seem to be most compatible with this therapy approach since the patient can easily practice structured drills (e.g., sustaining /a/ for as long as possible using loud phonation) over the telephone. Although some problems associated with this alternative method of service delivery (e.g., loss of selected frequencies and vocal characteristics during telephone transmission; methodologic problems in treating patients with hearing impairments), recent technological advancements such as the video phone are serving to increase the clinical applicability of this particular therapy approach.

An alternative solution for implementing in-clinic structured therapy programs involves the participation of speech pathology aides, nursing home staff, student volunteers, personal companions, or family members. These individuals can often be trained to work with patients on specific therapy tasks to increase the frequency of practice sessions. In addition to providing supplemental practice, this home programming strategy can greatly facilitate carryover of improved vocal behaviors to daily living.

Patients traveling a distance to receive therapy often benefit most from an intensive therapy program that includes two or more daily treatment sessions. Although this scheduling model seems particularly well suited for patients in need of short-term therapy to treat certain muscle misuse voice disorders such as conversion aphonia or mutational falsetto, other types of voice problems can also be effectively managed using this approach. For example, patients with vocal fold stiffness, unilateral vocal fold paralysis, and spasmodic dysphonias may be candidates for a 1- to 2-week intensive program of voice therapy that includes the development of a home-based vocal exercise program.

Among the therapeutic tools that can be successfully utilized in home programming are individualized video and/or audio tapes and visual or biofeedback devices. By recording selected segments of therapy sessions, a home practice tape can be generated which provides a review of recommended vocal exercises and procedures. Various types of visual or biofeedback devices, ranging from a portable surface EMG device to a sensory-powered Coca-Cola can or artificial flower that dances in response to the human voice (available in novelty stores), can also be used to enhance a patient's independent home practice. Self-help literature may also be employed selectively to guide appropriately motivated patients in home-based programs (e.g., Boone, 1991; Cooper, 1984; Lessac, 1967; Linklater, 1976; Rammage, 1996).

The Clinician

It is the clinician's responsibility to implement the selected procedures and monitor progress. The clinician's most serious task is to take into consideration all the physical, emotional, and environmental factors that can influence vocal pathologies and behaviors, and thus jeopardize therapy progress. When those considerations have been acknowledged and accounted for and the proper diagnosis ensured, the clinican can truly monitor patient progress.

Misdiagnosis sometimes occurs when one condition masks another during evaluation. For example, a small epidermoid cyst with associated edema may cause irritation on the contralateral fold, and this clinical presentation may be mistaken for bilateral vocal nodules. Voice therapy—instead of surgery—might be inappropriately recommended. Because behavioral therapy alone cannot eliminate a cyst, the therapy will ultimately prove to be unsuccessful due to misdiagnosis. By periodically monitoring the status of the vocal folds as a part of treatment, the clinician can often identify these types of problems. In the case of the epidermoid cyst, for instance, improved vocal hygiene and vocal abuse reduction might well decrease the surrounding edema and tissue irritation, thereby making the underlying cyst more visible with the aid of videostroboscopy.

Many patients have voice disorders that have multiple etiologies, so that diagnostic investigation must be an ongoing process in the therapy program. In a patient with chronic laryngitis, for example, the clinician may discover during the course of treatment that a combination of factors is serving to maintain the voice problem. One patient, a painter who was exposed on a daily basis to paint fumes and abusing his voice regularly during basketball practice was also taking Prozac® (fluoxetine HCI), an antidepressant which has a side effect of drying the laryngeal mucosa. His voice problems were resolved only when all three components of the disorder were addressed.

Effective planning and monitoring of voice therapy programs depends on astute direction by the voice clinician, who is constantly alert to the many variables that can influence human behavior and attempts at its intervention. The clinician's knowledge, experience, perceptions, judgments, and interpretations provide the necessary human-expert to direct a successful treatment program. The vocal function laboratory provides the means for the exact, objective measures of the efforts being made.

REFERENCES

Benninger, M. S., & Schwimmer, C. (1995). Functional neurophysiology and vocal fold paralysis. In J. S. Rubin, R. T. Sataloff, G. S. Korovin, & W. J. Gould (Eds.), *Diagnosis and treatment of voice disorders* (pp. 105–121). New York/Tokyo: Igaku-Shoin.

Bless, D. M. (1991). Assessment of laryngeal function. In C. N. Ford & D. M. Bless (Eds.), *Phonosurgery: Assessment and surgical management of voice disorders* (pp. 95–122). New York: Raven Press.

Bless, D. M., Ford, C. N., & Loftus, J. M. (1992). Role of injectable collagen in the treatment of glottic insufficiency: A study of 199 patients. *Annals of Otology, Rhinology and Laryngology, 101,* 237–246.

Blitzer, A., & Brin, M. F. (1992). Treatment of spasmodic dysphonia (laryngeal dystonia) with local injections of botulinum toxin. *Journal of Voice 6*(4), 365–369.

Blom, E. D. (1995). Tracheoesophageal speech. (Review). *Seminars in Speech and Language, 16*(3), 191–204.

Boone, D. R. (1991). *Is your voice telling on you?* San Diego: Singular Publishing Group.

Boone, D. R., & McFarlane, S. C. (1988). *The voice and voice therapy* (4th ed.). Englewood Cliffs, NJ: Prentice-Hall.

Brandenburg, J. H. (1980). Vocal rehabilitation after laryngectomy. *Archives of Otolaryngology, 106*(11), 688–691.

Brandenburg, J. H., Cragle, S. P., & Rammage, L. A. (1991). A modified neoglottis procedure: Update and analysis. *Otolaryngology-Head and Neck Surgery, 104*(2), 175–181.

Brandenburg, J. H., Kirkham, W., & Koschkee, D. (1992). Vocal cord augmentation with autogenous fat. *Laryngoscope, 102,* 495–500.

Brandenburg, J. H., Unger, J. M., & Koschkee, D. (1996). Vocal cord injection with autogenous fat: A long-term magnetic resonance imaging evaluation. *Laryngoscope, 106,* 174–180.

Christensen, L. B. (1977). *Experimental methodology,* Boston: Allyn and Bacon.

Colton, R. H., & Casper, J. K. (1990). *Understanding voice problems: A physiological perspective on diagnosis and treatment.* Baltimore: Williams & Wilkins.

Cooper, M. (1984). *Change your voice, change your life.* New York: Macmillan.

Crumley, R. L. (1991). Update: Ansa cervicalis to recurrent laryngeal nerve anastomosis for unilateral laryngeal paralysis. *Laryngoscope, 101,* 384–387.

Dedo, H. H., (1976). Recurrent laryngeal nerve section for spastic dysphonia. *Annals of Otology, Rhinology & Laryngology, 85,* 451–459.

Dedo, H. H., & Behlau, M. S. (1991). Recurrent laryngeal nerve section for spastic dysphonia: 5- to 14-year preliminary results in the first 300 patients. *Annals of Otology, Rhinology & Laryngology, 100,* 274–279.

Dedo, H. H., & Izdebski, K (1983). Problems with surgical (RLN section) treatment of spasmodic dysphonia. *Laryngoscope, 93,* 268–271.

Ford, C. N., (1991). Laryngeal injection techniques. In C. N. Ford & D. M. Bless (Eds.), *Phonosurgery: Assessment and surgical management of voice disorders.* New York: Raven Press.

Ford, C. N., & Bless, D. M. (1986). Clinical experience with injectable collagen for vocal fold augmentation. *Laryngoscope, 96,* 863–869.

Ford, C. N., & Bless, D. M. (1991). *Phonosurgery: Assessment and surgical management of voice disorders.* New York: Raven Press..

Gould, W. J., Rubin, J. S., & Yanagisawa, E. (1995). Benign vocal fold pathology through the eyes of the laryngologist. In J. S. Rubin, R. T. Sataloff,, G. S. Korovin, & W. J. Gould (Eds.), *Diagnosis and treatment of voice disorders* (pp. 137–151). New York/Tokyo: Igaku-Shoin.

Isshiki, N. (1989). *Phonosurgery: Theory and practice* (pp. 137–151). Tokyo: Springer-Verlag.

Karnell, M. P. (1991). Adjunctive measures for optimal phonosurgical results: The role of voice therapy in phonosurgery assessment and surgical management of voice disorders. In C. N. Ford & D. M. Bless (Eds.), *Phonosurgery: Assessment and surgical management of voice disorders* (pp. 213–224). New York: Raven Press.

Koshkee, D. L. (1991). *Treatment Efficacy Response Form.* Madison: University of Wisconsin Hospital and Clinics.

Koschkee, D. L. (1992, July). *Probe therapy.* Paper presented at the Second Biennial Phonosurgery Symposium, Madison, WI.

Koufman, J. A. (1986). Laryngoplasty for vocal cord medialization: An alternative to Teflon. *Laryngoscope, 96,* 726–731.

Koufman, J. A. (1988). Laryngoplastic phonosurgery. In J. T. Johnson, A. Blitzer, R. H. Ossoff, & J. R. Thomas (Eds.), *Instructional Courses, American Academy of Otolaryngology-Head and Neck Surgery, 1,* 339–350.

Kotby, N. (1994). *The accent method of voice therapy.* San Diego: Singular Publishing Group.

Lessac, A. (1967). *The use and training of the human voice.* New York: Drama Book Publishers.

Linklater, K. (1976). *Freeing the natural voice.* New York: Drama Book Publishers.

Ludlow, C. L. (1990). Treatment of speech and voice disorders with botulinum toxin. *Journal of the American Medical Association, 264*(20), 2671–2675.

Ludlow, C. L. (1995). Management of the spasmodic dysphonias. In J. S. Rubin, R. T. Sataloff, G. S. Korovin, & W. J. Gould (Eds.), *Diagnosis and treatment of voice disorders* (pp. 436–454). New York: Igaku-Shoin.

Ludlow, C. L., Bagley, J., Yin, S. G., & Koda, J. (1992). A comparison of injection techniques using botulinum toxin injection for treatment of spasmodic dysphonia. *Journal of Voice, 6*(4), 380–386.

Ludlow, C. L., Naunton, R. F., Fujita, M. & Sedory, S. E. (1990). Spasmodic dysphonia: botulinum toxin after recurrent nerve surgery. *Otolaryngology—Head and Neck Surgery, 102*(2), 122–131.

Ludlow, C. L., Naunton, R. F., Terada, S., & Anderson, B. J. (1991). Successful treatment of selected cases of abductor spasmodic dysphonia using botulinum toxin injection. *Otolaryngology—Head and Neck Surgery, 104*(6), 849–855.

Morrison, M., & Rammage, L., with: Nichol, H., Pullan, B., May, P. & Salkeld, L. (1994). *The management of voice disorders.* London: Chapman & Hall Medical & San Diego: Singular Publishing Group.

Ramig, L. O., Bonitati, C. M., & Horii, Y. (1991). The efficacy of voice therapy for patients with Parkinson's disease. *National Centre for Voice and Speech Status and Progress Report, 1,* 61–86.

Ramig, L. O., Bonitati, C., M., Lemke, J. H., & Horii, Y. (1994). Voice treatment for patients with Parkinson disease: Development of an approach and preliminary efficacy data. *Journal of Medical Speech-Language Pathology, 2*(3), 191–209.

Ramig, L. O., Bonitati, C. & Winholtz, W. (1994). *Lee Silverman voice treatment. A treatment video tape.* Denver: National Centre for Voice and Speech.

Ramig, L. O., Countryman, S., Thompson, L. L., & Horii, Y. (1995). Comparison of two forms of intensive speech treatment for parkinson disease. *Journal of Speech and Hearing Research, 38,* 1232–1251.

Rammage, L. (1996). *Vocalizing with ease: A self-improvement guide.* Vancouver: Pacific Voice Clinic.

Robbins, J., Fisher, H. B., Blom, E. D., & Singer, M. I. (1984). Selected acoustic features of tracheoesophageal, esophageal, and laryngeal speech. *Archives of Otolaryngology, 110*(10), 670–672.

Rubin, J. S., Sataloff, R. T., Korovin, G. S., & Gould, W. J. (Eds.). (1995). *Diagnosis and treatment of voice disorders.* New York/Tokyo: Igaku–Shoin.

Shulman, S. (1993). Symptom modification for abductor spasmodic dysphonia. In J. Stemple (Ed.), *Voice therapy: Clinical studies* (pp. 128–130). St. Louis: Mosby-Year Book.

Singer, M. I., & Blom, E. D. (1980). An endoscopic technique for restoration of voice after laryngectomy. *Annals of Otology, Rhinology and Laryngology, 89,* 529–533.

Stemple, J. (1993). Stemple-Barnes-Briese vocal function exercises. In J. Stemple (Ed.), *Voice therapy: Clinical studies.* St. Louis: Mosby-Year Book.

Takenouchi, S., & Matsu, T. (1971). Pedicled nerve muscle graft for recurrent laryngeal nerve paralysis. *XIII Congress International Bronchoesophagologie Societé* (pp. 225–227). Lyon, France: Sines Editions.

Tucker, H. M. (1977). Reinnervation of the unilaterally paralyzed larynx. *Annals of Otology, Rhinology and Laryngology, 86,* 789–794.

Tucker, H. M. (1988). Rehabilitation of the immobile vocal fold: Paralysis and/or fixation. In M. P. Fried (Ed.), *The larynx: An interdisciplinary approach* (pp. 191–202). Boston: Little, Brown.

Tucker, H. M. (1992). Combination surgical therapy for spasmodic dysphonia. *Journal of Voice,* 6(4), 355–357.

APPENDIX 6–1

Postoperative Patient Instructions

1. VOICE REST: For the first 48 hours following surgery you are to be on voice rest. This means that you are not to use your voice unless it is absolutely necessary, and when it is necessary, restrict your speaking to no more than five minutes within any one-hour period. Any talking should be soft, in a quiet environment, and in the middle of your vocal range where it is easiest to speak without strain. Do not engage in vocal throat-clearing or coughing. DO NOT WHISPER. Use a notepad, "magic slate," or other writing tools to communicate your needs. Cancel all social engagements. Stay at home and get plenty of rest and hydration. You can determine whether you are adequately hydrated by observing your urine: it should be pale in color; if it is dark and concentrated, you should increase your intake of non-caffeinated, non-alcoholic beverages.

2. RESTRICTED VOICE USE: For the week following 48 hours of voice rest, use your voice minimally. When speaking, you should be close enough to your listener to touch his/her shoulder. Do not engage in throat-clearing or coughing. DO NOT WHISPER. Do not speak outside, in groups, in a vehicle, airplane, or any other noisy environments, such as restaurants. Any voice use should be soft, in a quiet environment, and in the middle of your vocal range where it is easiest to speak without strain. During this period of restricted voice use, be sure you are adequately hydrated by drinking at least 8 glasses of non-caffeinated, non-alcoholic beverages daily.

3. PRUDENT VOICE USE: For the next two weeks before you return for your follow-up exam, you have few restrictions in your voice use. Observe common-sense rules of vocal hygiene. Avoid vocally-abusive activities: yelling, cheering, screaming, throat-clearing, coughing, loud or prolonged laugh.

Adapted from Bless, D. M. (1992). University of Wisconsin Hospital and Clinics, Madison.

CHAPTER

7

CLINICAL PROGRAM DEVELOPMENT

In today's competitive health care marketplace, successful clinical practice depends not only on the delivery of quality services to patients, but also on a number of other programmatic factors, such as implementing effective marketing strategies and collecting sufficient revenues to develop and maintain quality voice care programs. This chapter presents an overview of four facets of clinical program management that can impact on service delivery:

Clinical voice laboratory development,

Caseload expansion,

Marketing services, and

Reimbursement considerations.

CLINICAL VOICE LABORATORY DEVELOPMENT

The establishment of a clinical voice laboratory is important for several reasons:

▶ It is the arena in which theories of voice production are clinically applied to the evaluation process through objective documentation and interpretation of instrumental measures.

▶ Vocal function testing aids in establishing differential diagnoses and documenting baseline function.

▶ Instrumental analysis assists in treatment planning and improves clinical accountability.

▶ The information gained through instrumental assessment can enhance patient counseling and facilitate sharing of information within the voice care team.

Most experienced voice care professionals would agree that vocal function testing should be an integral part of all voice evaluations, but there are several practical reasons why this does not always happen. Clinical voice laboratories are not always available to practitioners and the creation of such a laboratory requires careful planning, financial support, knowledgeable personnel, technical assistance, and regular maintenance. Proper safety and hygiene precautions must be observed and adequate physical space must be allotted to house the clinical laboratory and its instruments. Any or all of these factors can be responsible for discouraging the practitioner who has not been previously involved in establishing a clinical voice laboratory.

New Area of Involvement

Only in recent years have clinicians been responsible for setting up instrumental laboratories. Consequently, the majority have little or no experience in this area. Yet, the growing number of clinical voice laboratories developing throughout the continent is testimony to the fact that practitioners recognize the importance of including instrumental evaluation as a part of their assessment batteries. Some common issues that need to be addressed are equipment needs and acquisition, clinical space acquisition, teaching and research accommodation, safety and hygiene, funding, maintenance, and user friendliness.

Surveying the Needs of the Medical Setting

In the preliminary stages of clinical voice laboratory development, it is advisable to determine the needs and goals of the medical setting with respect to new technology and instrumentation. Considering the needs of the institution, practitioners, patients, and the laboratory itself are all important aspects of a needs assessment survey.

Institution Needs

The justification for a voice lab requires an understanding of the goals and priorities of the medical center, its missions and administrative structure, and the methods and philosophical bases on which decisions about capital equipment funding are made. A review of the center's written policies and procedures and discussions with hospital administrators/clinic managers can provide valuable insights into the processes by which the institution introduces new technology into its operations.

Depending on current policies, procedures, and politics, it is generally possible to develop laboratory justifications that fulfill the needs of the medical setting. Table 7–1 identifies some of the most common needs, wants, and/or goals of institutions. For example, if a particular institution needs to improve its finances, a payback plan could be generated to demonstrate the cost-effectiveness of the equipment requested. If improving the quality of existing services is a priority, documentation that supports the use of instrumental testing as an accepted evaluation technique could be beneficial. Bless, Hirano, and Feder (1987); Woo, Colton, Casper, and Brewer (1991); Sataloff et al. (1988); and Faure and Muller (1992) have documented the diagnostic value of videostroboscopy. Literature is also available to support use of electroglottography (Baken, 1992; Gerratt, Hanson, & Berke, 1987; Hanson, Gerratt, & Ward, 1983; Karnell, 1989; Scherer, Gould, Titze, Meyers, & Sataloff, 1988) and electromyography (Kotby, Fadly, Madkour, Brakah, Alloush, & Saleh, 1992; Haglund, 1973; Luschei & Hoffman, 1991; Miller, 1992; Schaeffer, 1991). Manufacturers and vendors of clinical voice laboratory equipment can offer additional references.

Practitioner Needs

Examining the needs and activities of the practitioners who will work in the laboratory can help clarify the intended purposes of the facility. Sataloff (1991) points out that, although it is possible to develop a clinical voice lab that will be used exclusively for patient service, laboratories are often used for both clinical and research activities. In teaching hospitals, where both the institution and practitioners share an additional commitment to teaching, all three types of professional activities will likely exist.

Table 7–1 delineates some of the potential benefits of clinical voice laboratory devel-

TABLE 7–1. Needs assessment. Goals and benefits for development of a clinical voice laboratory.

Medical Setting Components	*Potential Benefits*
Institution	Quality assurance
	Increased revenue
	Improved competitive advantage
	Diversification of new services
	Expansion of existing services
	Support for referring physicians
	Reduced maintenance costs
	Improved safety and hygiene
	Support for clinical staff
Practitioners	Quality assurance
	Improved diagnostic methods
	Expanded treatment techniques (e.g., biofeedback training)
	Increased research capabilities
	Improved eligibility for grant funding
	Access to state-of-the-art technology for clinical teaching
	Increased incentive for interdisciplinary research teams/study groups

opment for practitioners. Naturally, the types and degrees of involvement in each area will vary with the interests, educational backgrounds, and experiences of individual staff members.

Patient Needs

Determining the needs of patients is an important consideration that must not be overlooked at any stage of voice laboratory development. By becoming familiar with the incidence of voice disorders and the availability of voice care services in the community, the development team can define the scope of practice needed to ensure quality patient care. Equipment selection and physical-environment planning are facilitated by identifying the types of patients to be seen, including unique characteristics of the patient populations that necessitate special accommodations.

Bless (1992) has discussed the importance of considering patient demographics as a part of the equipment selection process. She encourages clinicians to examine patient variables such as age, sex, diagnosis, physical limitations, and vocal capabilities because diverse populations may have special equipment needs. Examples include the need for smaller laboratory instruments to examine children, instruments with greater phonation ranges for professional voice users, and multipositioning examination chairs for nonambulatory patients.

Similarly, physical and environmental factors such as laboratory size, width of doorways, and access to running water cannot be ignored. In one unfortunate situation, clinicians were dismayed to learn that the entryway to their newly remodeled laboratory would not accommodate the extra-wide wheelchairs used by many of their patients with ALS.

Finally, in assessing patients' needs, consideration should be given to the availability of similar services within the community, as well as the potential for program growth, given the area's population and size. As Bless (1992) indicates, areas that are heavily populated with professional voice users (e.g., large cities, university towns with music schools and staff) are usually prime sites for developing or expanding voice care services. In other settings it must be determined that there is an adequately large population base to justify acquisition and use of the laboratory's technology.

Laboratory Needs

In determining the equipment needs of either a proposed or existing voice laboratory, it is customary to begin with an inventory of available items. Whether those items are previous purchases or equipment on loan from other departments, the inventory must account for replacement of valued instruments that are not functioning satisfactorily.

In general, when equipment is more than 7 years old, it is time to consider replacement. However, age alone usually does not justify replacing older pieces of equipment that do not have a history of excessive repairs. Maintenance costs should be calculated to determine whether the cumulative total exceeds the cost of replacement, or whether a single repair will cost more than one-half the replacement cost. Under either circumstance, it is probably more efficacious to replace the equipment.

When the inventory has been completed and decisions have been made about the replacement of necessary tools, the acquisition of new technologies will likely be considered. In equipping a start-up laboratory, instruments are generally needed to provide laryngeal imaging and videostroboscopic capabilities, aerodynamic measures of mean flow rate, lung volumes, and air pressures, and acoustic measures of frequency and intensity. These measures are used routinely in assessing the majority of voice cases. Additionally, new clinical laboratories should have equipment for making audio and video recordings, and autoclaving equipment for sterilizing parts that come into patient contact.

In instances where a basic voice laboratory has already been established, purchase of additional instruments can broaden the range and scope of assessment and diagnostic services, and make specialized diagnostic testing possible. Examples of equipment commonly requested by practitioners in well-established voice laboratories include:

▶ sophisticated acoustic analysis instrumentation/software: for example, instruments providing sound spectrography, phonetograms, and measures of spectral noise and pitch and amplitude perturbation;
▶ instrumentation that provides measures of respiratory function, such as flow volume loops and abdominal and rib-cage movements and pressures;
▶ instrumentation measuring vocal fold contact area, such as electroglottography; and
▶ equipment for neurophysiological evaluation, such as laryngeal EMG instruments.

Decisions about instrumentation needed for evaluation ultimately depend on the nature of the disorders represented in the patient population being served and the measures needed for accurate diagnosis.

Financial Planning

Securing funding for the purchase of biomedical instruments is the next major step in the equipment acquisition process. For those who are unable to obtain financial backing from an institution, a variety of funding options are available, for example, fundraising activities or federal and private sector grants. Without question, however, the most direct way of funding a voice laboratory is through the medical center's capital equipment procedure.

Although reimbursement structures and policies may vary among medical settings, most institutions regard purchase of equipment costing $1,000 or more as capital expenditures, and require submission of proposals that detail information about costs, needs justification, intended use, and item description and specifications. Subscribing to the institution's capital equipment application guidelines is almost always worth the effort.

Demonstrating the cost-effectiveness of new instruments is one way to justify equipment acquisition. For example, if it can be shown that a videostroboscopic system will more than pay for itself within 3 or 5 years, most administrators will agree that the institution's money is being well spent.

Some manufacturers have developed payback plans illustrating how the purchase price of their respective videostroboscopic systems can be regained through patient remuneration. The positive cash flow generated each month will repay the initial capital investment over time. Payback time can be projected based on the number of patients seen for evaluation each week and the cost of the evaluation service.

Another accepted financial planning technique that can be a useful adjunct to the justification process is a life-cycle cost analysis. This method uses calculations of the total cost of a project, including the initial capital cost, the operating costs for the expected lifetime of the equipment, and the time cost of the money.

In situations where cash flow is a vital concern, the option of leasing can be explored as an alternative to making a direct capital expenditure. Although system prices and lease programs tend to vary among companies providing voice laboratory instruments, many companies now offer leasing programs that include buy-out options at the end of the leasing term. Vendors typically have a variety of terms for their leasing programs, and can provide written documentation that identifies the advantages of leasing to assist in budget justification (e.g., potential tax breaks, fixed monthly payments, preservation of credit lines, conservation of business capital).

In some instances where only partial funding is available through the medical institution, and where the equipment will have multiple applications (e.g., clinical services, teaching, research), funding may be sought from several relevant sources that will use the system.

Equipment Selection

Because of the recent increase in available technologies, clinicians now have many more equipment options from which to select their specific diagnostic and assessment tools. Selecting the most appropriate laboratory instruments often involves representatives from several fields, including clinical engineering, infectious disease, nursing, and information processing, and well as the voice care team.

The process typically begins with efforts to gain greater knowledge about the specific types and brands of commercially available equipment. Voice care professionals can learn about laboratory instrumentation through conferences or workshops, networking with colleagues in similar medical settings, and reviewing the literature for relevant information.

Once a list of instruments and vendors has been acquired, clinicians can invite selected vendors to bring their products to the clinic for an in-house demonstration. This common practice enables the entire team, including equipment maintenance personnel, to make comparative evaluations.

In evaluating the overall suitability of instruments, a number of factors should be considered. Four basic principles are applicable to the equipment selection process: features, specifications, compatibility, and operating costs.

Cost Versus Essential Features

Since no single instrument or brand is necessarily the best choice for all clinical laboratories, a variety of makes and models should be examined. For example, it might be determined that a relatively inexpensive stroboscope, with all the essential components, is a reasonable choice for a program just beginning to offer videostroboscopic services. In constrast, a well-established clinical practice may decide to upgrade to a system with more auxiliary features, to improve efficiency and ease of testing. Upgrading to a more efficient, durable, or sophisticated unit can be particularly important in clinics with high-density patient populations (i.e., where 10 or more voice evaluations might be performed in a day) or where equipment is being used for multiple purposes.

A decision to purchase less expensive equipment does not necessarily mean compromised quality. In some cases, as in the stroboscope example, the sacrifice in terms of operation in a lower priced system may relate only to the loss of auxiliary features (e.g., digitized imaging, computerized file storage and retrieval, automatic tape recueing) rather than actual loss of laryngeal image quality. While these ancillary features are unquestionably assistive to clinicians, the trade-off in cost may be necessary in some situations.

Equipment Specifications

The purchasing team must carefully review the equipment specifications for requested items to determine that the instruments are capable of analyzing and/or conditioning signals within required ranges. Using guidelines for minimum and maximum range requirements can ensure that all comparable equipment meets agreed-upon standards (Table 7–2).

Equipment Compatibility

When new pieces of equipment are integrated into an existing laboratory set-up, or when individual components are combined to create a new or expanded instrumental system, all the equipment must be compatible. The most costly instruments available can obliterate quality control if they are not compatible with other components. If equipment compatibility is an issue, the purchasing group should consult their electronics technician and the manufacturer for specific recommendations.

Long-Term Operating Costs

Equipment costs do not end with the purchase price alone. Depending on the sophistication, complexity, and individual components of each instrument, as well as particular manufacturer/vendor policies, equipment operating costs can vary widely.

Because the costs of maintaining a particular instrument can influence equipment selection (usually in a case where two instruments are considered to be comparable in other respects), it is advisable to enquire about five major aspects of operating costs:

Initial Warranty: The purchasing team must check the length and terms of the manufacturer's warranty. Most standard warranties cover repair or replacement of

TABLE 7–2. Recommended equipment specifications for selected measures.

Measure	Units	Minimum	Maximum
Airflow rate	ml/sec	10	2,000
Air pressure	cm H$_2$0	1	30
Air volume	ml	100	6,000
Duration	msec	.001	60,000
Frequency	Hz	50	1,500
Intensity	dB SPL	50	120

any defective part or instrument within a 12-month period.

Extended Maintenance Contracts: The availability and costs of extended maintenance contracts should be clearly spelled out. These contracts, which provide continued maintenance and repair coverage for a specified period following expiration of the initial warranty (e.g., 2 years), are usually available only at the time of the original equipment purchase and may offer different levels of protection. Whereas an "all-inclusive maintenance package" might cover all costs associated with equipment maintenance and repair (e.g., labor, travel, system adjustments, cleaning, lubrication, software upgrading), a "limited-maintenance agreement" would cover only specified components, parts, and labor.

Because extended maintenance contracts are essentially insurance policies that ensure proper functioning of equipment over time, there are no hard and fast rules for deciding whether or not to purchase one. Like other insurance policies, the costs of insurance coverage must be weighed against a number of other factors: for example, the length of time the equipment has been on the market, its maintenance reputation, general structural integrity (durability), anticipated weekly usage, and overall contribution to the functioning of the clinical voice lab.

Software Upgrades: The equipment selection process must account for the need to upgrade software, particularly if plans for an upgrade are currently pending. As new features are added and newer versions are introduced, the purchasers need to know if software upgrades are included as a feature of the manufacturer's extended maintenance program.

Hardware Repairs and Modifications: Those responsible for maintenance should determine how repairs and modifications of equipment are managed (e.g., modifying a dedicated device so it can be interfaced with a computer). Increased clinic "down time" and lost patient revenues can be po-

tential problems, particularly in instances where the equipment has to be returned to its manufacturer in another country. The purchasing team should check on the customary turn-around time for repair of equipment at the manufacturer's site.

Expendable Supplies: The manufacturer should provide information about the types and costs of expendable supplies and replaceable parts that are necessary for optimal operation of the product. Because the prices of certain items may vary considerably (e.g., halogen and zenon bulbs), a more expensive unit can actually be made to appear more desirable to an administrator concerned with long-term operating costs. More commonly, however, it is evident that overall expenses are higher for "better" equipment. For example, high-grade videotapes might be essential for capturing the finest laryngeal images with a sophisticated videostroboscopic unit, so this extra expense should be committed at the outset to assure the system operates at optimal level.

Safety and Hygiene

As our medical settings have become increasingly dependent on technology, the potential risks to patients and practitioners have expanded proportionally. Observation of appropriate infection control and laboratory safety precautions can effectively nullify any risks to patients or staff in the clinical voice laboratory, but only if the procedures are practiced consistently by all professionals involved.

Several safety and hygiene guidelines can serve as a quick reference for busy practitioners, highlighting key components of a voice laboratory safety program:

General laboratory precautions (Table 7–3)

Procedures for disinfecting a rigid endoscope (Table 7–4), and

Guidelines to ensure electrical safety in the laboratory (Table 7–5)

TABLE 7–3. General laboratory safety precautions.

Wash hands immediately before and after any examination, even when gloves are worn.

Wear disposable surgical gloves (latex or other appropriate material) during every examination.

Use other types of personal protection devices (e.g., eyewear, face masks, gowns) to prevent any direct exposure to blood and other body fluids.

Avoid putting contaminated objects/used instruments directly on work surfaces.

Wash work surfaces regularly, using a suitable disinfectant.

Discard single-use products after one use.

Clean and disinfect instruments immediately after use.

Follow manufacturers' instructions for disinfecting/sterilizing equipment.

Use only disinfectants that are still active. Most disinfecting agents remain active for approximately 28 days after preparation.

TABLE 7–4. Rigid endoscope disinfecting procedure.

Clean and disinfect endoscopes immediately after use.

Rinse the working end of the endoscope by holding it under running water for 3–6 seconds.

Immerse approximately 3/4 of the working end in a disinfecting solution specified by institutional standards. An endoscope caddy works well for holding the endoscope in the germicidal solution.

Soak the endoscope for the minimum period of time specified by the manufacturer's instructions. Avoid oversoaking, as this can shorten the lifespan of the endoscope by loosening glue agents, clouding lenses, etc.

After disinfecting, rinse the endoscope well under running water to remove any residual germicidal solution that might irritate patients' tissues.

Air dry or wipe dry with a soft disposable tissue.

TABLE 7–5. Electrical safety measures.

Inspect new equipment before using for physical damage. Have required electrical and mechanical safety testing completed before using new equipment.

Retest all biomedical instruments periodically to ensure that they are performing safely, reliably, and accurately.

Use regular preventive maintenance (e.g., cleaning, lubricating, system calibration) to help eliminate hazards before they develop.

Minimize instrument abuse by familiarizing clinic staff with each instrument's operation and limitations.

Ensure that all electrical outlets are properly grounded. Have a technician check the laboratory's wiring if necessary.

Never use an adaptor to plug a three-pronged cord into a two-pronged outlet: the third contact on the outlet is the grounding component.

Space and Environment

One of the basic prerequisites for developing a clinical voice laboratory is acquiring adequate space. In some medical environments, space may not be a concern. In other settings, the lack of available space can be the foremost obstacle to voice lab development and expansion. In either scenario, it is advantageous to carefully plan the space allotted to maximize its usage, to ensure reliable testing conditions, to facilitate patient-clinician interaction, and to provide comfortable examining conditions.

According to Bless (1992), a laboratory facility must be at least 10 × 12 feet to accommodate its basic functions and permit routine diagnostic testing. This assumes that videostroboscopic, aerodynamic, acoustic, and other basic voice function tests will take place in the same room. There are several advantages to such an arrangement:

▶ it creates a standardized testing environment for different measures;
▶ it minimizes patient "traffic" and disruption of the assessment process; and
▶ it makes simultaneous measures possible, in cases where this is desirable

Additional space would likely be required for performing special evaluation procedures (e.g., EMG studies, which necessitate space for a bed or cot), storing confidential patient files (e.g., computer disks, video/audiotapes), and housing supplemental biofeedback (therapy) equipment.

Another important consideration is to create an acoustic environment that will allow the production of high-quality recordings. If the voice lab itself is not suitable for this purpose, a nearby ancillary room (e.g., a sound booth or sound shelter) needs to be secured.

Finally, the laboratory environment should be made to appear uncluttered and efficient, yet unintimidating. Visual and auditory distractions should be minimized, for example, by attenuating extraneous noise and concealing equipment cords. If a second video monitor is placed so patients can observe their own larynxes during the videolaryngoscopic evaluation, they can participate more actively in the testing situation as required. The ambience should be as comfortable as possible so patients can relax and provide reliable and valid responses. When invasive procedures, such as laryngeal EMG are being conducted, or in cases where patients are anxious, soft background music or engaging videotapes can provide effective distractions as long as they do not interfere with the testing procedure or results.

CASELOAD EXPANSION

Expanding a clinical program's services and caseload is dependent on a well-conceptualized plan, good public relations, high standards of patient care, and a resourceful administration. Defining and prioritizing the types of new or expanded clinical programs that are needed or desired is a first step. Table 7–6 lists some services that are commonly marketed in program expansion.

The success of service expansion may depend on the program's internal and external visibility. In the medical setting, administrators, medical staff, support staff, and other professionals all need to be educated about the types of services being provided. Through public relations efforts, potential referral sources outside the hospital or clinic can be made aware of unique benefits offered by new or expanded programs.

A number of promotional tools are available to assist in this process (refer to Marketing of Services).

The level of patient care and "customer satisfaction" is the single strongest promotional influence, because satisfied patients are a primary referral source. It is important to recognize that quality care begins, not with the initial evaluation, but with patients' first contact with the clinic. Therefore, the roles of the scheduling secretary and receptionist are keys to program expansion. If patients are treated respectfully

TABLE 7–6. Common markets for caseload expansion.

DIAGNOSTIC SERVICES:
Videostroboscopic Studies
   Laryngeal function

Videoendoscopic Studies
   Laryngeal function
   Velopharyngeal function
   Esophageal function

Videofluoroscopic Studies
   Swallowing function
   Esophageal function
   Laryngeal function

Vocal Function Studies
   Vocal/laryngeal function

Nasal Function Studies
   Velopharyngeal function

INDIVIDUAL TREATMENT PROGRAMS:
Cancer patients
   Patients with laryngeal cancer
   Patients with oral or naso-pharyngeal cancer

Patients with neurological dysfunction
   Patients with neurological diseases: Parkinson's disease, dystonias, ALS, MS, etc.
   Patients with traumatic brain injury: CVA, MVA, etc.
   Tracheotomy/Ventilator-dependent patients
   Professional/Occupational voice users
   Pediatrics
   Geriatrics
   Patients with hearing impairments

BIOFEEDBACK THERAPY:
Patients with VCD/paradoxical vocal fold movements
Patients with specific muscle misuses
Patients with velopharyngeal dysfunction

VOICE CARE WORKSHOPS:
Vocal performers: singers, actors, broadcasters, etc.
Occupational voice users: teachers, clergy, lawyers, sales representatives

SUPPORT GROUPS:
Cancer patients
Patients with spasmodic dysphonias
Patients with neurological disease: Parkinson's, dystonia; etc.
Patients with congenital anomalies

during initial telephone encounters, scheduled for appointments within a reasonable period of time, and provided with adequate information about clinic location, parking, registration procedures, insurance preauthorization, and other preparatory information, they usually feel more positive about the evaluation experience.

Additional factors that may influence patients' perceptions and ratings of service include their reception on arrival (patients want to feel expected and welcome), the waiting time before being seen for an evaluation (more than 20 minutes is too long), the cooperative spirit and communication among team members (patients often silently observe and evaluate the interchanges between professionals), follow-up with the referral source (patients legitimately expect that written reports will be generated promptly and sent out to referring physicians as well as others to whom they have released information), and follow-up with the patient (e.g., scheduling any follow-up appointments needed, phone contact after an evaluation to determine if there are any questions about the results or recommendations).

The administrator's role is also key to caseload development for several reasons. First, financial planning or backing is often required for developing new or expanded clinical programs. Second, a skilled administrator can assist clinicians in identification of existing and underserved client bases, remaining current in their marketing approaches, and long-range planning. Third, the administrator can help implement successful billing procedures and revenue collection, a process that ultimately determines whether or not a clinic is financially viable.

MARKETING OF SERVICES

Marketing is "the process of planning and executing the conception, pricing, promotion, and distribution of ideas, goods, and services to create exchanges that satisfy individual and organizational objectives" (American Marketing Association, 1985, p. 1). "Central to this definition of marketing is the focus on the consumer, whether that be an individual patient, physician, or organization such as a company contracting for industrial medicine. This definition also contains the key ingredients of marketing that lead to consumer satisfaction. Increasingly in health care, customer satisfaction is the key issue" (Berkowitz, 1996). Rynne (1995) further highlights the consumer-focus of marketing in his definition: "Marketing is the science and art of understand-

ing how humans make choices, how to respond to those choices, and how to influence consumers' choices" (p. 7). When applied to the "business" of voice care, these definitions can guide administrators, clinicians, voice teachers, and other professionals who are involved in determining marketing objectives and strategies.

A wide range and scope of promotional tools and activities can be used to inform consumers about the availability of services (Table 7–7). Assessing the effectiveness of particular strategies is essential.

One helpful approach for assessing the viability of specific marketing techniques is to perform a referral-base analysis before and after implementing selected marketing activities. This method documents any changes in referral patterns that might result from marketing efforts. In the example provided (Table 7–8), there were increases in the number of referrals received from physicians in gastroenterology, following a series of marketing activities that promoted voice care services during the month of February. Of course, to make use of this type of referral tracking mechanism, the source of every referral must be determined, either through patient questioning or written history intake information.

REIMBURSEMENT CONSIDERATIONS

One of the most common questions asked by patients during initial clinic contacts is: "Will my insurance cover the charges?" (Quam, 1994, personal communication). The prevalence of this question is both understandable and revealing. Most patients are clearly concerned about the potential impact of recent increases in health care costs on their coverage of health care services.

Voice care professionals can assist patients with the reimbursement process by following several basic guidelines:

▶ **Provide patients with medical billing codes when requested.**

TABLE 7–7. Marketing strategies.

Marketing Tools	Marketing Activities
Brochures	In-Services:
Business cards	Music department/groups
Newsletters	Theater department/groups
	Medical/Allied Health groups
Reports	Conference presentations
Written reevaluation reminders	Community presentations
"Thank-You" letters to referral sources	Support-group meetings
Educational pamphlets	Health fairs
Yellow pages ads	TV/Radio/Newspaper interviews
Magazine ads	Screening programs
	Personal contacts with key people
	Outside consultations
	Follow-up phone calls with patients
	Communications with third-party providers
	Consumer satisfaction surveys

TABLE 7–8. Voice clinic referral-base analysis.

	Total Number of New Patient Evaluations			
Referral Source	JANUARY	FEBRUARY[1]	MARCH[2]	APRIL[3]
External referrals	8	0	7	8
Internal referrals	31	30	38	40
General medicine	9	6	9	8
Neurology	6	6	5	6
Pulmonary	7	8	6	8
Gastroenterology	2	3	8	9
Pediatrics	5	6	6	5
Gerontology	1	0	2	2
Endocrinology	1	1	2	2
Total	39	37	45	48

[1] 1 month of marketing campaign to Gastroenterology.

[2] 2 months following marketing campaign to Gastroenterology.

[3] 3 months following marketing campaign to Gastroenterology.

Although health care providers are generally not in a position to counsel nor even reassure patients who are anxious about their insurance coverage, they can often facilitate the preauthorization process by identifying the professional diagnostic and treatment codes that will be used for billing. Because insurance carriers rely heavily on medical billing codes to determine whether particular procedures are included in their insurance plan benefits, insurance representatives frequently require information about "expected" medical billing codes before they will advise patients about whether or not services are likely to be covered.

In the USA, CPT codes, or Physician's Current Procedures terminology, provides "a listing of descriptive terms and identifying codes for reporting medical services and procedures." The use of CPT coding is now standard practice in medical settings in the USA, and is essential for third-party reimbursement. New editions of CPT codes are issued annually. Because new editions generally contain many revisions, it is critical that updated codes be submitted on reimbursement forms to expedite claim processing. In Canada, each province issues annual provincial fee schedules that provide medical billing codes and standardized fees for specified procedures.

▶ **Refrain from giving fee estimates.**
In general, it is best to allow billing personnel to quote estimated fees when they are required. Although some practitioners feel as if they are doing patients a favor by providing fee information, they may actually be doing a disservice in cases where inaccurate or outdated fee information is given, or when there are additional questions about billing or insurance coverage (e.g., deductibles, co-payments). Instead, the clinician should be prepared to identify a contact person in the hospital or clinic who can fully answer patients' questions about fees based on the designated medical billing codes.

▶ **Use ICD-9-CM codes properly.**
Another coding system, the ICD-9-CM or International Classification of Diseases-9th Revision-Clinical Modification—Fourth Revision (1995), is used for reporting medical diseases and diagnoses. Like CPT codes, ICD-9-CM codes are required for third-party reimbursement.

Because diagnosis code selection can sometimes influence a patient's eligibility for coverage, it is wise to stay informed about the current rules and regulations for using codes, particularly Medicare codes, because they are often used as a standard for other insurance carriers. For example, one of the diagnoses currently covered by Medicare is hoarseness (ICD-9-CM: 784.89), an appropriate diagnosis code for use with an elderly patient coming into the clinic with a complaint of "hoarseness" and presenting a hoarse voice and raspy voice quality. An alternative diagnosis for the same patient might be atrophic laryngitis (ICD-9-CM: 476.0). Although use of this latter code would also be an appropriate diagnostic choice, it might well result in claim rejection because it is not one of Medicare's reimbursable diagnoses.

The issue here is for professionals to be knowledgeable enough about code usage that they can work with the system to minimize claim rejections and maximize reimbursement. Naturally, intentional abuse of codes is unacceptable and legally constitutes fraud.

▶ **Provide statements of medical necessity.**
Statements of medical necessity are written statements that are prepared and signed by the health care provider, indicating that the expenses incurred for the treatment have been prescribed to treat, alleviate, cure, mitigate, or prevent a specific medical condition. If treatments are prescribed to improve a patient's general health and well-being or for cosmetic purposes, they are not considered medically necessary.

Health care professionals are regularly asked to write letters to insurance providers stating that the recommended medical treatments are deemed to be "reasonable, necessary and appropriate" given the patient's condition. Typically, these letters need to provide information regarding the patient's diagnosis, onset, and severity of symptoms, prior treatments, and a rationale for the treatment.

▶ **Direct patients toward "hotline" assistance sources.**

Should patients encounter reimbursement problems, there may be assistance for some just a phone call or web-line away. For example, Allergan Inc. has established a toll-free reimbursement hotline to assist patients with spasmodic dysphonias deal with reimbursement problems related to botulinum toxin treatments.

▶ **Generate reimbursable reports.**

The information provided in the clinical report may be accurate and supportive of reimbursement by insurance agencies, or accurate and unsupportive of the recovery of voice care expenses. Hospital adminstrators can play an essential role in helping the voice care team generate reports that legitimize the patient's claims to the insurer. By taking care to represent the patient's problem and justify necessary procedures using standardized and recognized terminology and codes, the report writer generates a guideline for the insurer that can be accepted and acted on most expediently and definitively.

▶ **Reassure patients that medical care is a right.**

The patient will be most receptive to proposed treatments if he or she believes that the cost is manageable. Although technology has given us the means to assess and treat patients more effectively than ever before, it has done little to increase the accessibility of services. Coverage and reimbursement gaps are an integral component of today's dynamic health care environment. In the current climate of "managed care," marketing and advocacy activities are more important than ever. Any extra efforts required on the part of health care workers to ensure that needed care is accessible and legitimate medical expenses are supported by exisiting insurance programs should not be considered extravagant or futile.

CONCLUSION

Advances in our understanding of vocal physiology and pathology, as well as technological developments, have launched voice care professionals into an era where comprehensive and sophisticated patient management is possible. The most formidable challenge that confronts practitioners attempting to implement current knowledge and technology is the dynamic medical climate: we find ourselves working in a system that is characterized by ongoing economic and political flux and constraints.

The daily involvement of the voice care team in advocacy activities supporting vocal health is no longer an altruistic choice, rather it is a moral *and* professional obligation. During an era when universal health care is not a reality, and the health care system is in constant transition, the voice care team needs to maintain "an active voice" to ensure continuity of the essential health care service it provides and to nurture the scientific growth that will advance this medical specialty into the twenty-first century.

REFERENCES

American Marketing Association. (1985). AMA board approves new definition. *American Medical News, 15*(5), 1.

Baken, R. J. (1992). Electroglottography. *Journal of Voice, 6*(2), 98–110.

Berkowitz, E. N. (1996). *Essentials of health care marketing.* Gaithersburg, MD: Aspen Publishers.

Bless, D. M. (1992, July). *Voice lab essentials: The set-up, equipment options.* Paper presented at the Second Biennial Phonosurgery Symposium, Madison, WI.

Bless, D. M., Hirano, M., & Feder, M. D. (1987). Videostroboscopic evaluation of the larynx. *Ears, Nose and Throat Journal, 66.*

Faure, M.-A., & Muller, A. (1992). Stroboscopy. *Journal of Voice, 6*(2), 139–148.

Gerratt, B. R., Hanson D. G., & Berke, G. S. (1987). Glottographic measures of laryngeal function in individuals with abnormal motor control. In T. Baer, C. Sasaki, & K. S. Harris (Eds.), *Laryngeal function in phonation and respiration.* Boston: Little, Brown.

Haglund, S. (1973). *Electromyography in the diagnosis of laryngeal motor disorders.* Stockholm: Boktryckeri AB Thule.

Hanson, D. G., Gerratt, B. R., & Ward, P. H. (1983). Glottographic measurement of vocal dysfunction: A preliminary report. *Annals of Otology, Rhinology and Laryngology, 92,* 413–420.

International Classification of Diseases (9th rev. Clinical Modification 4th rev., Color Coded) (1996). Los Angeles: Practice Management Information Corporation.

Karnell, M. P. (1989). Synchronized videostroboscopy and electroglottography. *Journal of Voice, 3*(1), 68–75.

Kotby, M. N, Fadly, E., Madkour, O., Barakah, M., Alloush, T., & Saleh, M. (1992). Electromyography and neurography in neurolaryngology. *Journal of Voice, 6*(2), 159–187.

Luschei, E., & Hoffman, H. (1991). Use of electromyogram (EMG) as a diagnostic aid for voice disorders. *National Centre for Voice and Speech Status and Progress Report, 1,* 129–150.

Miller, R. H. (1992). Technique of percutaneous EMG-guided botulinum toxin injection of the larynx for spasmodic dystonia. *Journal of Voice, 6*(4), 377–379.

Rynne, T. J. (1995). *Healthcare marketing in transition.* Los Angeles: Richard D. Irwin, A Times Mirror Higher Education Group, Inc.

Sataloff, R. T. (1991). *Professional voice: The science and art of clinical care.* New York: Raven Press.

Sataloff, R. T., Spiegel, J. R., Carroll, L. M., Schiebel, B. R., Darby, K. S., & Rulnick, R. (1988). Strobovideolaryngoscopy in professional voice users: Results and clinical value. *Journal of Voice, 1*(4), 359–364.

Schaefer, S. D. (1991). The treatment of acute external laryngeal injuries. "State of the art." *Archives of Otolaryngology—Head and Neck Surgery, 117,* 35–39.

Scherer, R. C., Gould, W. J., Titze, I. R., Meyers, A. D. & Sataloff, R. T. (1988). Preliminary evaluation of selected acoustic and glottographic measures for clinical phonatory function analysis. *Journal of Voice, 2*(3), 230–244.

Woo, P., Colton, R. D., Casper. J. K., & Brewer, D. (1991). Diagnostic value of stroboscopic examinations in hoarse patients. *Journal of Voice, 5*(3), 231–238.

INDEX